STRENGTH TRAINING

FOR

LONGEVITY

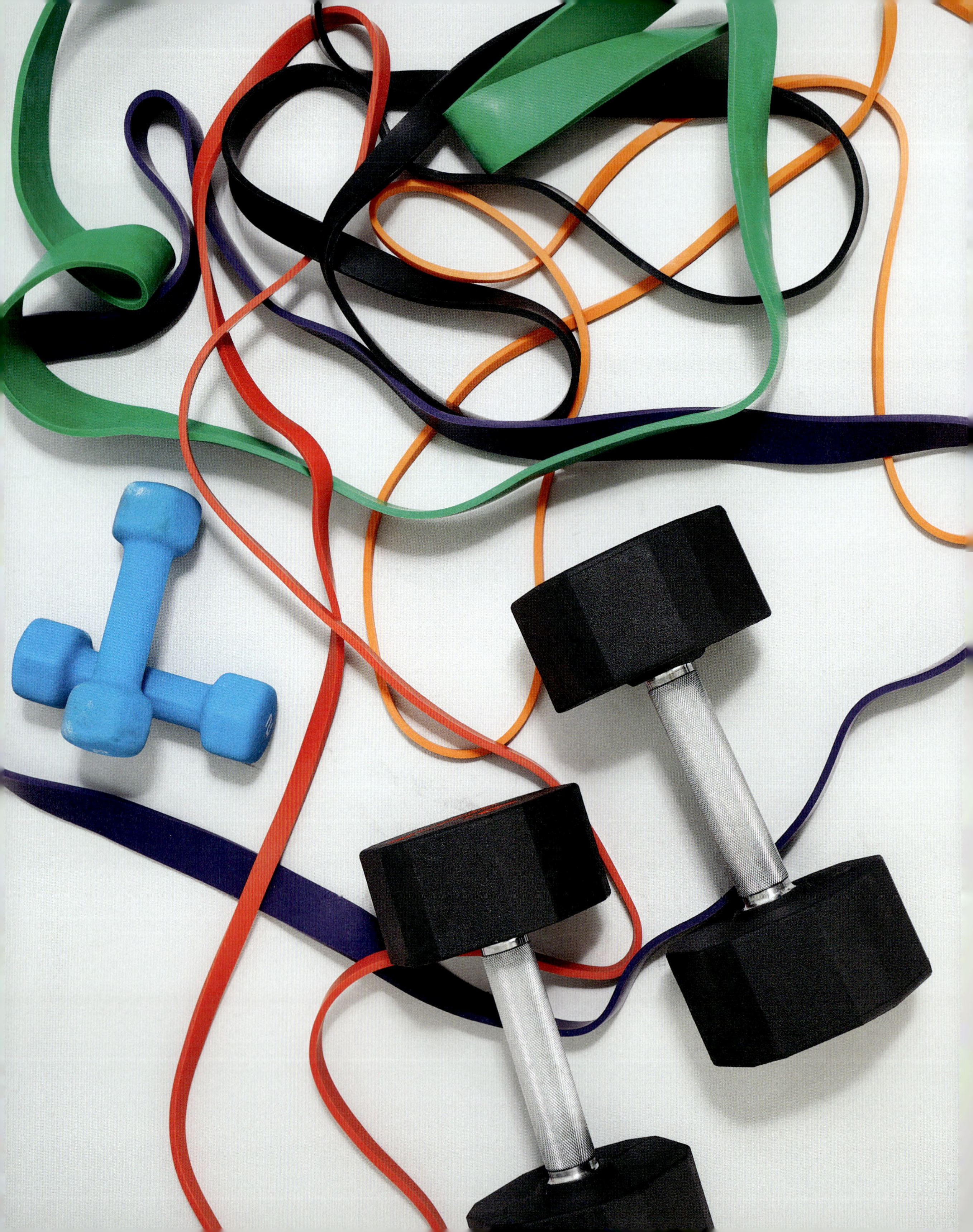

STRENGTH TRAINING
FOR
LONGEVITY

Simple Workouts for a Lifetime of Health and Mobility

Matt Schifferle

Photographs by Jena Cumbo

ZEITGEIST • NEW YORK

Zeitgeist™
An imprint and division of Penguin Random House LLC
1745 Broadway, New York, NY 10019
zeitgeistpublishing.com
penguinrandomhouse.com

ISBN: 9798217331031
Ebook ISBN: 9798217331024

Printed in the United States of America
1st Printing

Photographs © by Jena Cumbo
Hair and makeup by Sara Jade
Design by Katy Brown
Edited by Sarah Curley

The authorized representative in the EU for product safety and compliance is Penguin Random House Ireland, Morrison Chambers, 32 Nassau Street, Dublin D02 YH68, Ireland. https://eu-contact.penguin.ie

To my grandpa, Elmo Schifferle,

who taught me that simple habits

are the key to adding years to life

and life to those years

Contents

Lower Body *76*

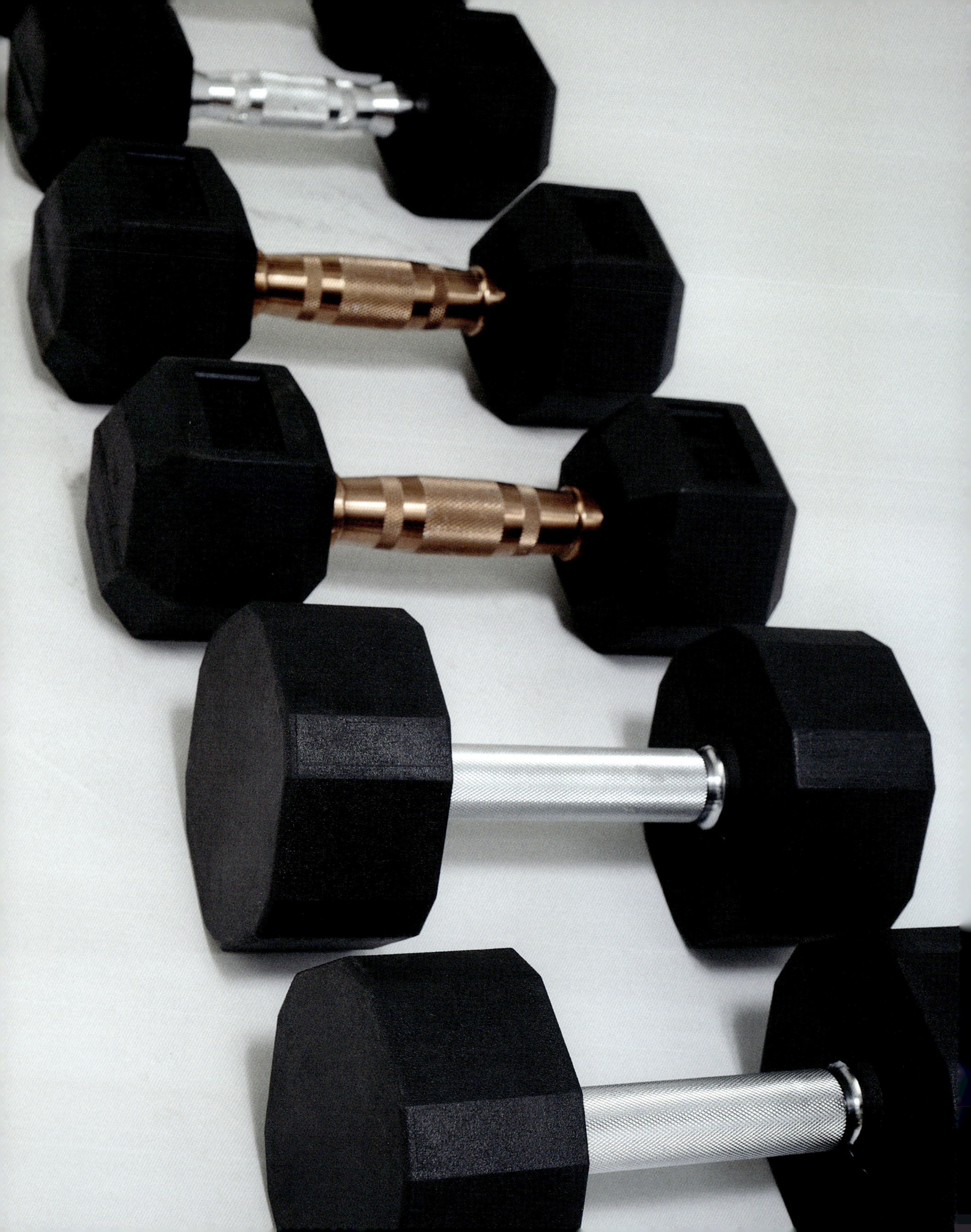

Introduction

Do you remember how great you felt when you were younger? How strong, mobile, and resilient you were? Like you could bounce back from anything life threw at you. I hope so, because I don't have many of those memories.

As a kid, I was always sick and achy. My poor joints protested even modest physical activity. Somehow, my body missed the memo that being young was supposed to protect me against physical affliction.

Thankfully, as a teen, I discovered physical training. I trained in martial arts, cycling, and outdoor sports and then started weight lifting. All of these disciplines made me stronger, healthier, and more resilient—at first. Over time, these pursuits broke me down. Martial arts burned me out and crushed my motivation. Endless cardio training made me stiff and injury-prone. Weight-lifting programs left me feeling beat-up, rather than healthy and strong.

It wasn't until I reached middle age that I learned strength training can be a potent form of medicine when approached correctly. I became a professional fitness coach and spent years working to achieve the proper training dose and approach—one that promotes longevity rather than compromises it. Now I teach folks just like you, through personal training and books I write, how to use strength training to achieve longevity.

Whether you're new to exercise or seeking a new regimen, this book can help you build overall strength and vitality for both the short and long term. This book is unlike other texts on strength training because it's about building more than just brute strength and muscle—it's also about developing holistic physical qualities through strength-training programming and habits that can add both years to your life and life to your years.

How to Use This Book

We'll start by exploring the fundamental elements of strength training and why they're essential for building lifelong resilience. I'll explain the different techniques and methods and the role they'll play in your success. Some techniques may be familiar; others new. You may find new ways to apply old techniques, and sometimes this is the best way to discover new levels of your potential. And if this is all new to you, you'll benefit from all this information!

Next, I'll show you how to apply these tools and techniques through a simple and efficient plan that's adaptable to your personal fitness level and abilities.

To start, just read through this book and get an overall feel for the information. You don't need to read it like a novel; feel free to focus on sections that offer new ideas and insights, and skim the parts that are already familiar.

Before you start your program, spend time setting up your equipment and trying out the various exercises. You don't need to create a perfectly optimized routine from day one. Play around and get a feel for the exercises as a way to introduce your body to the techniques. When you're ready, use the templates provided (page 49) to plan how you'll apply these techniques in a structured routine that works for you.

Whether you're new to exercise or seeking a new regimen, this book can help you build overall strength and vitality for both the short and long term.

Setting Expectations and Tips for Success

No one has ever won a race in the first leg, but countless people lose their race during the first leg. Why? Well, they start out going too fast, burn themselves out, or break their body and spirit. Here are some tips for managing expectations and long-term success:

Embrace the journey. Strength training for longevity is a journey that extends beyond the horizon. Start slow, set a manageable pace, and celebrate milestones as they come.

Notice the shift. You'll feel your body changing in subtle ways at first, like feeling stronger as you climb stairs or less stiffness when you get out of bed in the morning. Appreciate the progress as it happens.

Show self-compassion. Don't beat yourself up if life sometimes gets in the way. It's normal to skip a workout or fall off track from time to time. Just resume your training as soon as you can.

No one gets where they want to go by chasing perfection, and thankfully you don't need to. All that's necessary is to keep taking another step forward.

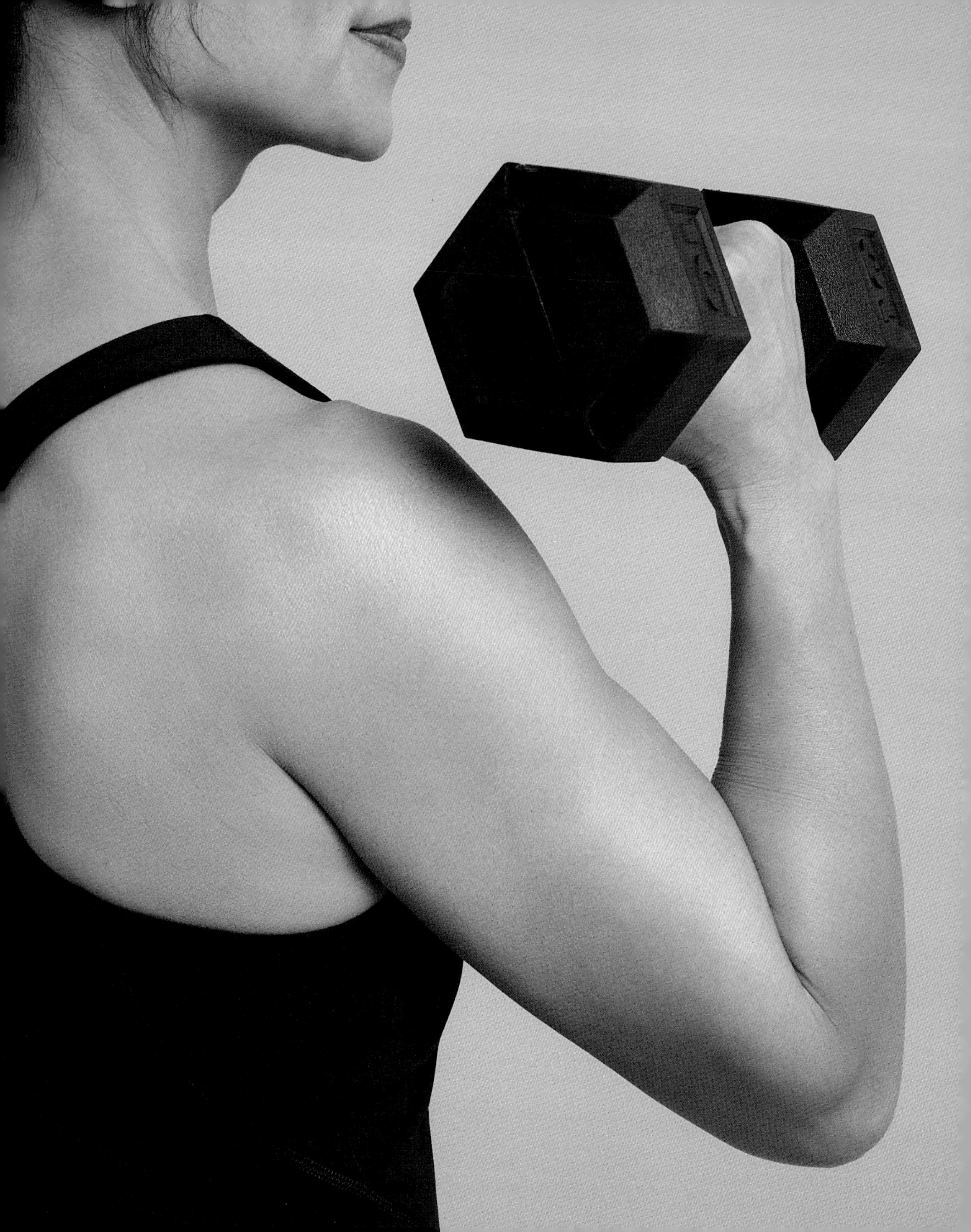

CHAPTER 1

Building Strength for the Future

The Core Principles of Longevity

The longevity of the body is heavily corelated to its ability to function well, especially as we age. Therefore, the principles of longevity are synonymous with the principles of physical functioning and capability.

Strength is the most fundamental principle in all physical functionality. The simple action of contracting your muscles is the foundation upon which all physical ability, and, therefore, longevity depends on.

Endurance is the next principle of longevity. This is the ability to use your strength for longer periods of time and resist fatigue.

Coordination is the use of your strength in the functional qualities necessary for stability, mobility and reducing stress on sensitive areas like the lower back.

This program is based on these principles. Using exercises that require coordinated strength, while challenging your endurance will maintain, and even build, your functional fitness which supports all aspects of your physical longevity.

What Is Longevity?

"Longevity" is a term that most everyone may understand, yet it can mean something different for each of us. For the athlete, longevity may mean being able to perform well throughout a season or enjoy a long career. A business owner may define longevity as the ability to conduct business with integrity and adhere to the founding principles of their company over several generations. But most of us will define longevity as being able to live longer while enjoying a high quality of life.

In every sense of the word, longevity boils down to achieving and maintaining beneficial qualities despite the inevitable challenges that occur over time. When it comes to fitness, a program designed for the long term is the cornerstone for living a healthy quality of life and promoting personal longevity. Unfortunately, this quality is often missing in our modern fitness culture, one in which so many bypass an active lifestyle in the interest of faster and more drastic results.

Let's explore the relationship between the sustainability of a fitness program and longevity of life.

Both anecdotal and scientific data paint a bleak perspective about the amount of time people enjoy the pursuit of a fitness regimen. Every New Year, people sign up for gym memberships that go neglected after a few weeks. Those who lose weight through trendy diets most often gain it right back. Even serious, self-motivated athletes often face injury and burnout, causing them to quit their fitness routines long before they get as far as their dreams and talents promised to take them.

The lesson is that the longevity of life and health is possible only with a fitness plan that promotes the longevity of your habits. You can only add years to your life if your habits are sustainable throughout those years. Prioritizing sustainability in your fitness plan is the key to achieving such results. Look at it as a shift in lifestyle rather than a plan with a finite beginning and end.

Research makes the importance of an active lifestyle crystal clear. Look at any long-term study on anything from weight loss to disease prevention, and even mental decline, and you'll find that sustainability is at the heart of success.

While all the research points this way, it's surprising how hard it can be for many people to put their good intentions into action that lasts. We all want to feel and look good, so why can't we get enough momentum going to stay the course and make the shift into a new lifestyle that will help us feel better and live longer?

We need to be able to envision the long game. To do this requires us to shift our life view and see ourselves prioritizing our health and longevity as fundamental goals that we honor each day. Sure, there will be days you don't feel well, or days packed end to end with other responsibilities, and you just don't get it done. That's okay. But if you get back in there the next day or week—as long as you're trying—you're making progress.

Unsurprisingly, you're more likely to stick with your exercise plan if you feel good. Longevity depends on many factors, as does our motivation to get up and do the work needed to stay strong. As you develop and maintain your strength-training program, learn as much as you can about the health habits that complement exercise to help you feel your best and live your best life:

Sleep: Sleep may feel like down time, but your body is busy at work repairing, restoring, and resetting bodily systems. Conversely, poor sleep habits are associated with increased short- and long-term health risks. Consistent and sufficient sleep serves a critical purpose in ensuring good health.

Nutrition: Like physical training, your nutrition habits can increase or decrease your longevity. That's why it's best to focus on the basics, like eating mostly whole foods, avoiding processed foods, and including a wide variety of colors and nutrients in your diet, with an emphasis on protein and plant-based foods. We'll explore this more later.

Habits for Longevity

- Hydrating
- Limiting alcohol and stress
- Living with gratitude and optimism
- Not smoking or quitting smoking
- Socializing

The Science Behind Strength Training

The human body has evolved over eons to become an ultra-efficient survival machine. Every aspect of physical fitness, from strength and power to strong bones and even coordination, is something our body will only hold on to if it's absolutely necessary. Once you stop telling your body to hold on to a capability, it will erode that ability to save variable physiological resources.

Prioritizing only the most necessary physical abilities suited our ancestors very well, but it doesn't bode well for our modern lifestyle. Long ago, it was impossible to do anything without physical activity. We couldn't eat, travel, socialize, or protect ourselves without physical activity. Now, we can accomplish all these things and still be productive members of society, with a fraction of the physical exertion necessary even a couple of generations ago.

A little lack of activity prompted our body to become more efficient. Now, we have so little activity that we aren't as efficient; we're weaker and frailer. And, as individuals, the less we do, the more we lose. This places us at a greater risk of illness, injury, and the detrimental effects that compromise our quality of life and our lifespan. We need physical activity to maintain the functional qualities that keep us healthy, and, yes, alive. The challenge is in finding practical methods through which to consistently produce such activity.

Because modern lifestyles are naturally more sedentary, people must make a greater effort to incorporate physical activity into their daily routines. Our busy lives often leave us with little time and energy, so how can we get a full day's worth of physical stimuli when we can't spend all day being active?

This is where proper strength training comes in. The nature of strength training is to subject the body to a style of physical activity that increases the intensity of demand upon the body. This increase in intensity means your body can experience a full day's worth of physical stimuli in a relatively short period of time.

Don't let the term "strength training" fool you. A proper training program will challenge far more than just the contractile force of your muscles. You'll also experience benefits in stability, mobility, cardiovascular stamina, endurance, coordination, and more. All these functional elements play a holistic role in your long-term health and fitness, in a single but comprehensive workout.

STRENGTH TRAINING IS FOR EVERYONE

Despite the many benefits of strength training, people are still hesitant, even stigmatized, by the concept. When I was growing up, you practiced strength training only if you were a serious athlete or a bodybuilder. Some well-meaning coaches even told me to avoid it, cautioning that it would make me slow and "muscle bound." Others openly discouraged strength training, claiming it was dangerous or not beneficial for certain demographics—those too young, too old, too skinny, too fat, too weak, and, yes, even too strong. I've heard 'em all—and they're all myths.

At its core, strength training isn't anything unusual—it's simply using your muscles regularly and intentionally. Technically, you engage in strength training every time you move your body or pick up something off the floor. The practical application of strength training is simply using the fundamental physical processes you already engage in every day in a more purposeful way.

This fundamental nature of strength training is what makes it effective for everyone. You already use your muscles on a daily basis, and your body is constantly adapting to the physical demand you place on your muscles with everything you do. Practical strength training is just using that process to your advantage. You don't need to qualify or be worthy of the benefits of strength training any more than you need to qualify to laugh with a friend or enjoy your favorite meal.

Like many, I once felt I wasn't strong enough or good enough to practice strength training. Here's the secret: The less qualified you feel you are to strength train, the more beneficial it is to you. The older you get, the more strength training can add years and vitality to your life. The less athletic and coordinated you are, the more physical ability you'll gain. The weaker and frailer you feel, the more strength training will make you resilient to stress.

It all comes back to the principle of "use it or lose it." The detrimental qualities that hold you back from strength training are the very things you'll alleviate through strength training. No one naturally has strength, vitality, coordination, or resilience. Everyone who possesses these qualities does so only because something they do, or have done, required them to have them. Strength training is nothing more than purposely pursuing the development of the very abilities you desire so you can build and maintain them to live your best life.

Fitness as the Foundation of Longevity

One of the biggest myths about strength training for longevity is that the benefits come just from getting stronger. Sure, strength is important, but there are plenty of "strong" people who are still frail and weak on the whole. In many ways, a singular focus on developing strength can make you less resilient.

In contrast, fitness for the sake of longevity is a holistic pursuit. Being able to contract your muscles is great, but you also need to be able to apply your strength for your overall functional benefit. This means you'll also need to develop coordination, mobility, and stability. Otherwise, you end up becoming "gym strong," able to do impressive things on a weight machine, but still struggle to climb a flight of stairs, or throw your back out picking up a sack of groceries.

These holistic qualities both depend on and promote strength. The more stable you are, the stronger you can become, and vice versa. Increased stability and strength help promote greater control and mobility, and the more mobile and coordinated you are, the easier it'll be to develop additional stability and strength.

It's this collection of physiological qualities that adds years
to your life and life to your years. More importantly, these are the
qualities that foster personal lifestyle independence. They ensure
that you have the physical ability to do the things you want to do,
especially as you get older. You can travel around the world without
worrying about physical limitations preventing you from climbing
a mountain or touring an ancient city. You can gain the confidence
and energy to play with friends and family in recreational activities.
This well-rounded approach to strength training will help you maximize your lifestyle potential, whatever that looks like for you.

MORE MOVEMENT

It's important to point out that strength training helps promote
healthy physical activity in other beneficial disciplines. Strength
training can be the cornerstone of your approach, but engaging in
other forms of sports and recreation will also deliver complemen-
tary benefits. Strength training ensures your body can handle the
physical demands of whatever supplemental activities you want to
enjoy so you can reap as much benefit and enjoyment from practicing them as you wish.

Don't feel limited by this list—what you choose to do may
depend on your location, physical abilities, or interests—just make
it something you enjoy!

Stay Active Beyond Workouts

- Boating (canoeing, kayaking, paddleboarding, rafting, sailing)
- Cycling
- Dance
- Hiking
- Pilates
- Skiing (cross-country or downhill)
- Social or team sports
- Swimming
- Yoga

Your Unique Approach to Strength Training

There are many different ways to approach strength training, and there's no single correct way to go about it. My approach is to incorporate various holistic elements in a simple and efficient manner to help you get the healthiest results with less time and effort.

Fitness Assessment

Let's start with a basic fitness assessment to get a baseline of your physical capabilities. This is important because you want to base your program off your personal abilities rather than blind assumptions about what might be best for your age or demographic. Complete and reflect on the following techniques to gauge your baseline.

Walk-and-Talk Test

This assessment tests overall stamina and cardiovascular endurance. You can perform this test outside or on a treadmill. The goal is to increase your walking pace or incline steadily until you find it a little challenging to walk and hold a conversation. This can be handy information for programming your workouts to be either more strength-based or more cardio-challenging.

Quality to look for

- How hard you can push your training pace and tempo before you start to experience a challenge to your cardiovascular system

Standing Overhead Reach

This first technique helps you assess your upper-body mobility and shoulder strength. Stand with arms at your sides, then rotate your arms in front of you in a semicircle to hold them straight up over your head.

Qualities to look for

- Your ability to hold your arms straight up overhead without your hands slightly in front of you
- Straight alignment in your torso without arching backward or moving your neck forward

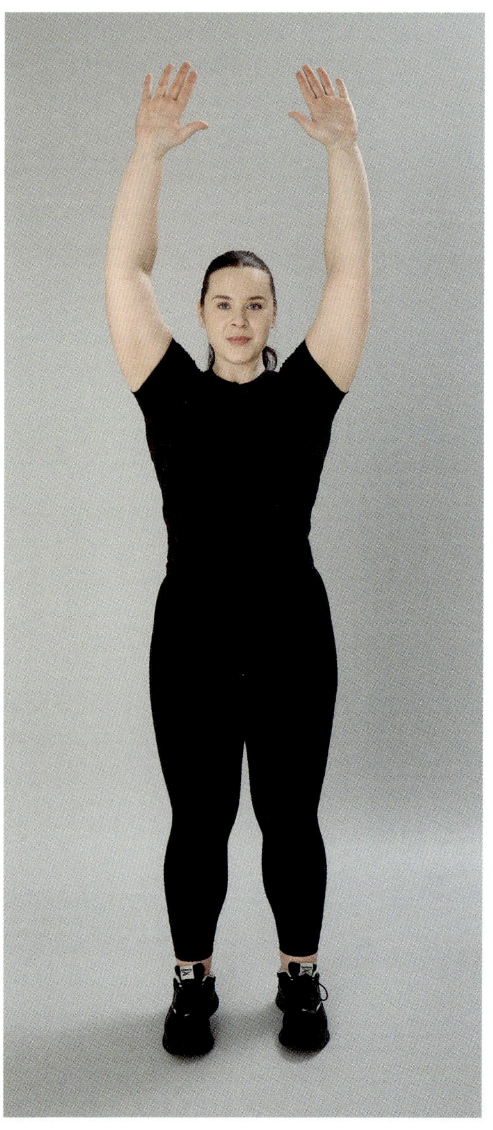

Single-Leg Stand

This is a basic stability and mobility assessment tool. You'll stand on one leg while you lift your other leg in a bend in front of you and hold.

Qualities to look for

- Your ability to stand with all of your weight on one leg without having to put the toes of the other foot on the ground
- The height you can lift the nonsupporting leg in front of you.

It's fine to place your hands on a countertop or a sturdy piece of furniture for support. Just make a note that you used some upper-body assistance.

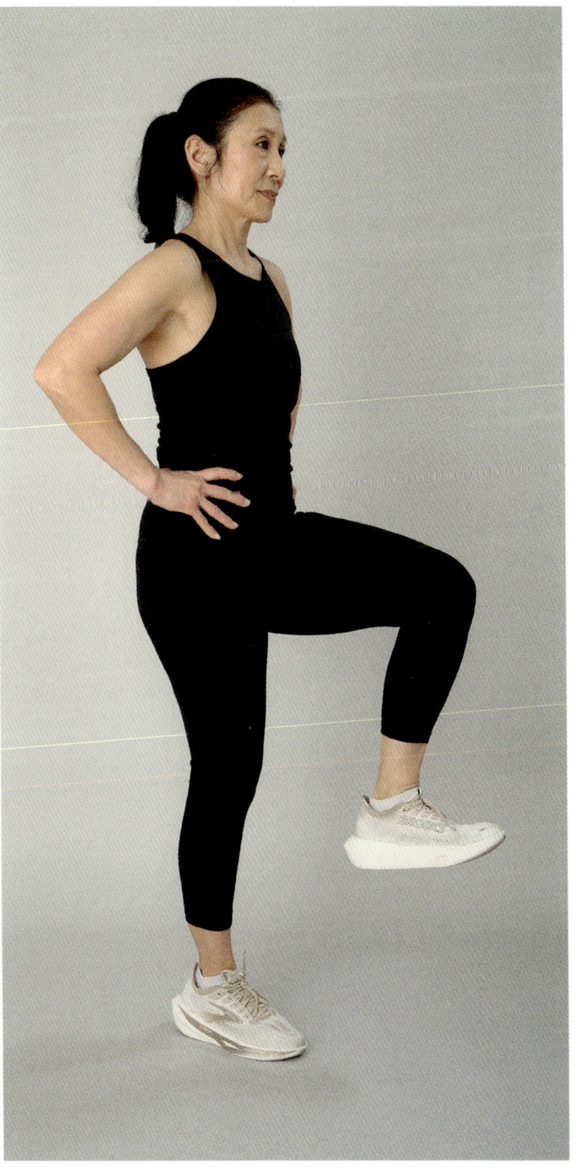

Plank Hold

This assessment technique looks at your upper body strength and core stability. Begin by placing your hands and feet on the floor in a push-up position, with arms straight. Hold your body in a straight line from shoulders to toes.

Quality to look for

- The ability to maintain a straight body without sagging your lower back or hunching your shoulders

If this is difficult, assume this position with hands on an elevated surface, like a sturdy piece of furniture.

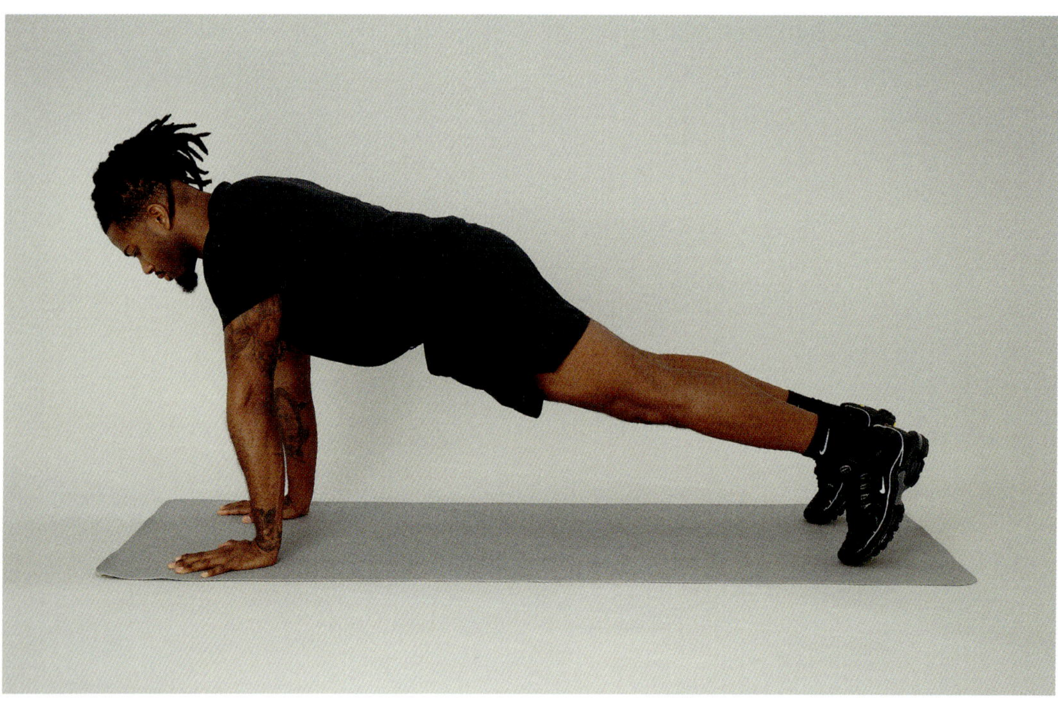

Squat Test

The squat test helps assess your lower-body strength, stability, and mobility. Lower yourself to sit back onto a chair or couch, then stand up without leaning forward too much. You can either hold your hands out for stability or drop them to your sides as you rise.

Qualities to look for

- The strength to lower your hips gently to the chair without falling back and letting your weight rest on your hips
- The ability to stand up without having to lean forward excessively or use your arms or armrests to help yourself up

To further test your lower-body strength, try to squat without using a chair. This tests your ability to hold and control yourself throughout your full range of motion.

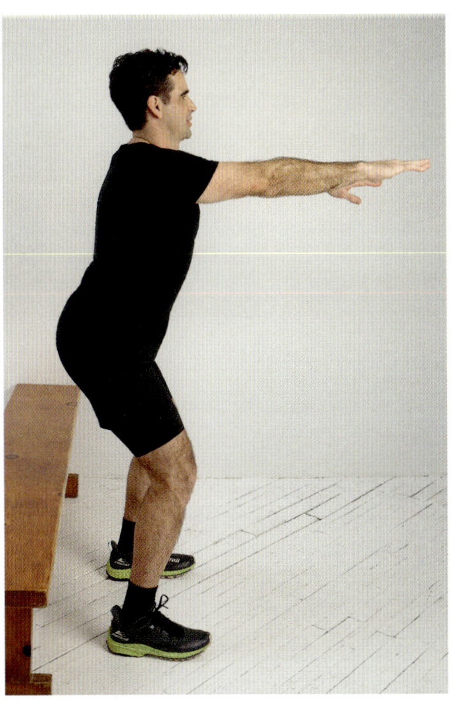
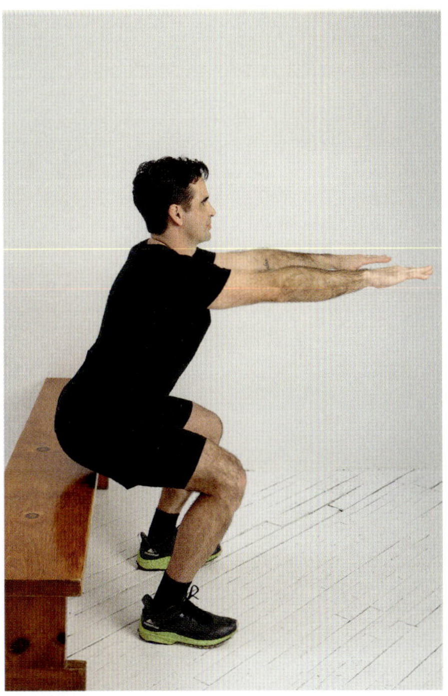

Hang Test

This test requires an overhead support like a doorway pull-up bar or equipment at a gym or playground. It's a basic shoulder mobility test that also assesses grip and back strength.

Qualities to look for

- The ability to hold yourself up with a good portion of your body weight on your hands (by transferring some weight from your feet to your hands)
- The ability to hold all of your weight by picking your feet up off the floor

If you don't have the strength to hold yourself off the ground, maintaining some of your weight on your feet can give you an assessment of how much weight and resistance you can pull with your hands.

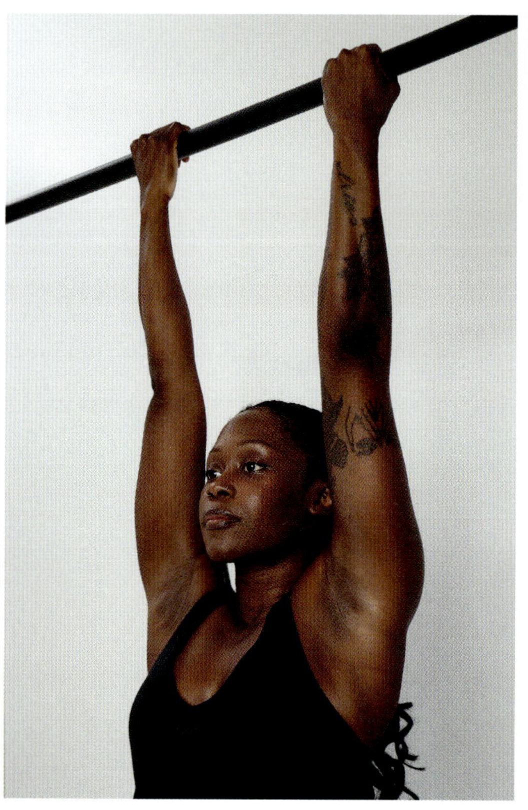

Equipment

With strength training, simple is best. This program uses just a few simple, cost-efficient tools in conjunction with basic fundamental exercises, providing exceptional benefit from a minimal investment.

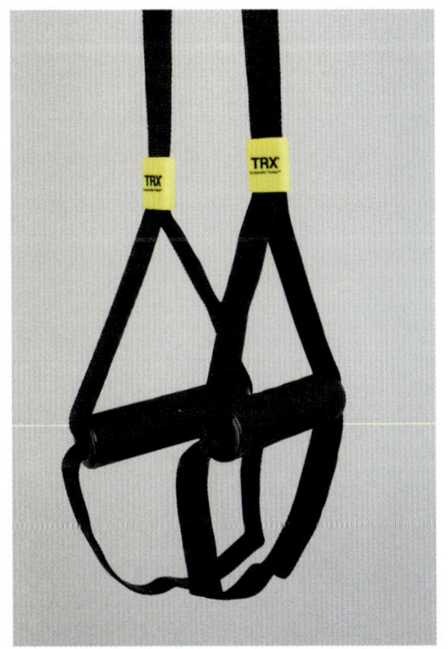

The most important thing to understand about strength training is that it's not about the tools you use, but how well you use your muscles. You may find certain tools work better for you with some exercises than for others. It's also okay not to use certain tools. Use what feels most comfortable and effective to you.

SUSPENSION STRAPS

Suspension straps are my all-time favorite piece of strength-training equipment. They create, essentially, a complete weight machine that fits in your pocket. You can use suspension straps anywhere, from the local gym to a bedroom or hotel room, by hanging them on a door through the included door anchor. Suspension straps give you control of how much resistance you're working with, simply by changing your body position.

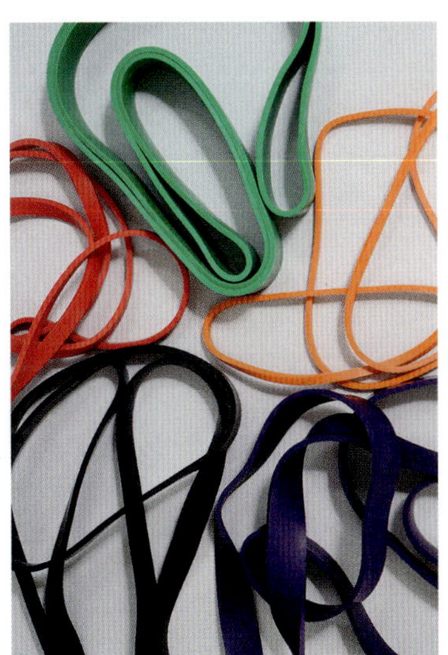

RESISTANCE BANDS

Resistance bands are another low-cost, portable strength-training option. Like suspension straps, resistance bands can be used with a door anchor to deliver resistance in a variety of directions. Many bands come with door anchors, or you can purchase one separately for about $5. I recommend having at least three bands to offer a range of resistance, including a light band you can stretch for 20 reps or more, a moderate band you can stretch for 10–19 reps, and a heavy band you can stretch for 3–9 reps.

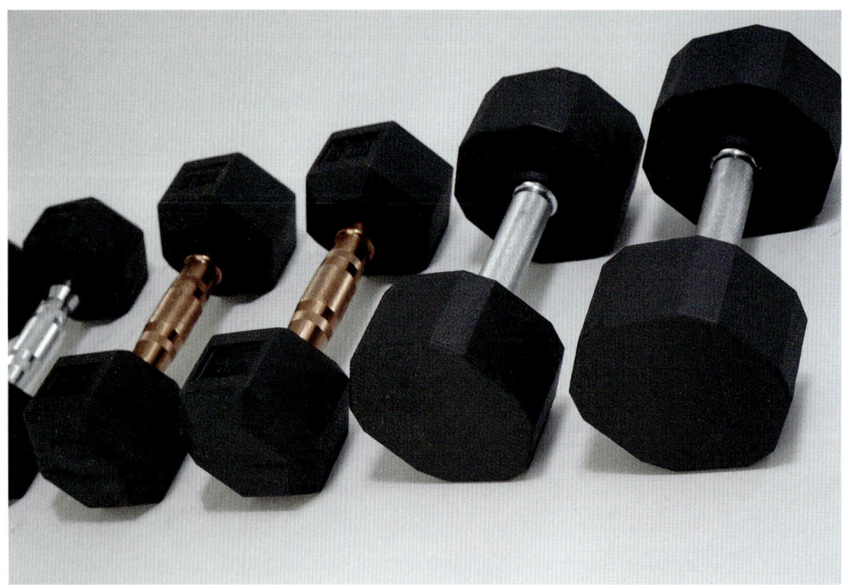

DUMBBELLS

Dumbbells are simple and versatile, and they work with your body. You don't necessarily need a full gym of hand weights; most people are fine with three or four selections that range from fairly light to pretty heavy. This might range from 3, 5, or 10 pounds to 35 or 40 pounds, depending on your abilities. You'll probably want heavier weights as you progress.

A STURDY SURFACE

A sturdy elevated surface is a useful piece of equipment, and it's something you've already got at arm's reach. This can be a sturdy chair, countertop, or couch. You may even find an outdoor ledge or park bench that suits your needs.

Long-Term Changes That Lead to Longevity

Like many disciplines in life, strength training only works if you can stick to it with relatively little effort over long periods of time. This is why it's important to make physical activity and strength training a daily habit, even if you practice it for just a few minutes at a time.

Technically, your body doesn't know what exercise is. All it understands is functional demand. Every moment of every day, your body constantly adapts to what you ask it to do. Asking your body to use strength, stability, and mobility on a daily basis will ensure that you build and maintain those qualities for a lifetime of benefits.

While the strength-training program in this book will provide you with life-giving vitality, you'll benefit even further by adopting a mindset that prioritizes daily movement. Walking is one of the easiest and most efficient ways to include longevity-boosting activity in your daily routine. Even small habits, like taking the stairs or parking your car a little farther away from the store, add up to benefit your overall health. Going for a short walk in the evening can also help you take a break from screens and reduce mental stress. Stress on your body, mind, and lifestyle is the single greatest threat to longevity, and reducing unproductive stress will do wonders for increasing your well-being and your chances of long-term success.

Nutrition Essentials

Health longevity is about much more than just strength, training, and exercise. Your ability to gain and sustain a higher level of health throughout your life is also greatly dependent on your diet.

This makes sense from a standpoint of basic inputs. You may engage in physical exercise a handful of times each week, but you make nutrition decisions many times every single day. The choices you make may seem trivial from one meal to the next, but their influences add up quickly for both positive and negative outcomes. Compound these outcomes over many months and years, and you see quickly why a healthy diet is essential for your long-term health.

THE IMPORTANCE OF PROTEIN

Protein is the cornerstone of a healthy diet, especially when it comes to health in longevity. Amino acids—the building blocks of protein—play a key role in nearly every physiological process responsible for your health and fitness.

Strength training naturally increases your daily protein require-ment by requiring more recovery after intense physical training. However, you don't necessarily need to be guzzling protein shakes and snacking on 32-ounce steaks just because you're practicing daily strength techniques.

Most active adult adults get plenty of protein at roughly 0.6 to 0.8 grams per pound (454 grams) of body weight. For a typical 150-pound individual, that would equate to 90 to 120 grams of protein per day. Naturally, your nutritional needs will increase the more active you are, as well as if you're trying to gain weight. Start with this amount as a rough baseline, and adjust your diet so you have steady energy levels throughout the day without feeling constant hunger or cravings.

A good general guideline to ensure adequate protein intake is to make protein the mainstay of each meal. Start by choosing a good protein source, then add plant-based foods and other sources of grains or carbohydrates to create a satisfying meal.

BUILDING A LONGEVITY-SUPPORTING DIET

Much of the common "healthy eating" dietary advice we hear in our fitness culture is actually counterproductive to longevity. Most fad diets prioritize restriction and deprivation under the assumption that your diet will become healthier as long as you eat less of certain "bad" foods.

It's an understandable assumption. Many people struggle with poor diets due to the overconsumption of processed fats, carbohydrates, and alcohol. However, a truly healthy diet isn't about restriction and deprivation, but rather satisfaction and fulfillment. A healthy diet feeds and supports your body, mind, and lifestyle. It gives you the nutritional building blocks to maintain a strong body and fuel a vibrant lifestyle. This objective is a lot easier to reach when your focus is on satisfaction instead of dietary restriction!

A truly satisfying diet for the long term is based on nutrient-dense wholesome foods; that is, foods that energize and strengthen all the different body systems. Note that "complete proteins" refers to proteins that contain all nine essential amino acids. On pages 34 and 35, you'll find a list of some of the more common whole foods that pack a powerful nutritional punch with their protein content as well as a variety of other nutrients and vitamins.

Snacking can have a place in a healthy diet, but in modern eating patterns it has become increasingly common, sometimes replacing regular, balanced meals. Meal preference is always an individual choice, but I've found it's easier to stick to a supportive, satisfying diet if you eat two or three full-size meals per day. Doing so makes it a lot easier to satisfy your nutritional requirements while also focusing on wholesome foods rather than quick processed snacks.

Some people like to snack before or after physical exercise. This can be helpful if you want a bit of fuel right before your workout—a piece of fruit or a granola bar can usually suffice. Likewise, eating after exercise can help stave off hunger, especially if you know your next meal is several hours away. In this case, a protein-rich option like a tuna sandwich or protein shake can satisfy your hunger and supply your muscles with valuable protein for recovery.

Protein-Rich Foods

ANIMAL SOURCES (COMPLETE PROTEINS)

- Chicken breast and thighs
- Cottage cheese
- Eggs
- Greek yogurt or skyr
- Lean beef (especially grass-fed)
- Salmon, sardines, mackerel
- Shellfish: shrimp, oysters, mussels, clams
- Tuna
- Turkey

VEGETABLE SOURCES (MICRONUTRIENT POWERHOUSES)

- Beets
- Broccoli
- Brussels sprouts
- Cabbage
- Carrots
- Cauliflower
- Collard greens
- Edamame
- Kale
- Red bell peppers
- Spinach
- Sweet potatoes
- Swiss chard and beet greens

Fiber- and Nutrient-Rich Foods

FRUITS (ANTIOXIDANTS AND PHYTONUTRIENTS)

- Apples
- Bananas
- Berries: blackberries, blueberries, raspberries, strawberries
- Kiwi
- Oranges and citrus
- Pomegranates

WHOLE GRAINS, BEANS, AND STARCHES

- Barley
- Beans: black, kidney, navy
- Lentils and chickpeas
- Oats
- Quinoa
- Rice: brown and wild
- Seeds: chia, hemp, pumpkin
- Sweet potatoes and yams
- Whole-grain bread and pasta (look for 100% whole grain on label)

HEALTHY FATS AND NUTS

- Avocados
- Flaxseed
- Nuts: almonds, cashews, pistachios, walnuts
- Oils: avocado and olive

EXTRAS: NUTRIENT "BOOSTERS"

- Bone broth
- Seaweed
- Fermented foods, like tempeh, sauerkraut, miso, kimchi, kefir
- Herbs and spices, like turmeric, parsley, ginger, garlic, cinnamon
- Nutritional yeast

However, don't feel like you "must" eat something just because you're engaging in physical activity. An exercise session may feel like it places a substantial demand on the body, but typically the increased need for nutrition it creates is relatively small.

Pay attention to your appetite and honor it as it fluctuates naturally. When you feel more hungry, by all means increase the portion size of your meals, or add an extra snack or two. But don't feel like you need to force-feed yourself. There's little need to add more food to your diet if you're satisfying yourself with several wholesome meals each day.

WHAT ABOUT SUPPLEMENTS?

Unless your health-care provider has ordered certain supplements for you, most supplements aren't critical when you consume wholesome, nutrient-dense foods. Supplementation from quality sources can help fortify your diet and fill in nutrients that may be in short supply. However, trendy supplements that promise radical results rarely deliver on their promises. Here are a few supplements worth considering as you embark on your strength-training journey.

Creatine: Creatine is one of the most studied and supported supplements, and we're still finding benefits from this cost-efficient supplement, which is helpful for energy production during high-intensity exercise.

Protein powder: Protein powder can help you meet your protein needs, especially if you have trouble getting a few solid meals in on a daily basis. Whey protein is the popular choice, but plant-based options, like pea protein, can help those who have issues with dairy.

Vitamin and mineral supplements: A simple vitamin pill is a standard—and for good reason. It's a bit of insurance for filling in gaps in your micronutrient needs. This is especially true for vitamins B12 and D, calcium, and iron.

Proper hydration plays an important role in everything from appetite regulation to physical performance. I recommend starting the day with something to drink, as you can lose water overnight while sleeping. It's also a good habit to keep a water bottle on hand throughout the day, especially while exercising.

Consistently getting some water throughout the day is generally more practical and helpful than worrying about how many ounces of water you're consuming. You don't need to force yourself to consume large amounts of water to adhere to some sort of guideline. If you go to the bathroom pretty frequently, you're likely more than meeting your hydration needs.

All About Recovery

Intense physical training can be stressful on the body, which makes recovery another important aspect of a healthy lifestyle. During recovery—the time between strength-training sessions—your body builds and repairs the damage that occurs during training. Your body also starts to adapt to ensure there's less damage the next time it's exposed to that stress.

A prominent example of this adaptation is muscle soreness. The first time you practice a new exercise, you may feel sore a day or two afterward due to the inflammation caused by the stress of the exercise. It can be uncomfortable, but your body will quickly adapt to the stress of that exercise. You'll notice you're not nearly as sore after the second time you practice that exercise because your body has adapted to handle the stress of the exercise with less damage, which plays a massive role in increasing longevity. This

Active Recovery Ideas

- Easy cycling or stationary biking
- Elliptical training
- Gentle flow yoga
- Light cardio to increase blood flow and break up inflammation
- Slow rowing or SkiErg training
- Swimming

adaptation makes the body more resilient to stress, so it doesn't break down as easily, and helps it recover faster when it experiences other forms of stress, such as illness or injury.

One of the biggest myths about recovery is that it requires complete rest for several days. You don't need 48 hours of down time just because you did a workout. In fact, you may recover faster by engaging in some light activity, sometimes known as "active recovery." The premise of active recovery is to move the body through some light and gentle movements that promote mobility and increase blood flow. Aim to engage your muscles and loosen any stiffness you may feel—just don't go so hard and long that you feel like it's turning into another workout. You want to finish feeling like you're just getting ramped up and ready to engage in more strenuous activity.

The most important thing about recovery is to give yourself as much time as needed rather than sticking to a dogmatic formula. The amount of recovery you need depends on how much stress and damage you experience from a workout, which is also influenced by your level of fitness, how harsh the training was, and other lifestyle factors, like sleep and diet. Generally, recovery between strength-training workouts takes two to three days to occur, but listen to your body. If you feel like you need more time to come back strong, give yourself that time. However, if you're ready to rock 'n' roll after even 24 hours, then give yourself the chance to continue.

Additionally, stretching and mobility exercises work to ease soreness and promote blood flow to working muscles. This type of mobility training is best if it requires some degree of work from the muscles.

Light strength work can also help break up inflammation and promote mobility, especially when practiced in a large range of motion. This effective form of active recovery

Active Recovery Activities

- Light shadow boxing or bag work
- Playing catch with a frisbee
- Shooting hoops
- Hitting balls at a driving range or playing a light round of golf

Make Time
for Mobility

- Deep squatting
- Holding stretches while also keeping the target muscles slightly tense
- Shoulder circles and standing twists

involves the same exercises you did for your workout, but with less resistance and intensity. For example, if you were doing resistance band pull-downs, use a lighter band than you used for the workout, and perform twice as many reps. The goal is to increase blood flow through the muscle but not work it hard. You want to make the muscles feel warm, but not burn. Use as much range of motion as possible to stretch out the stiff or sore muscles. The muscles should feel refreshed afterward rather than tired.

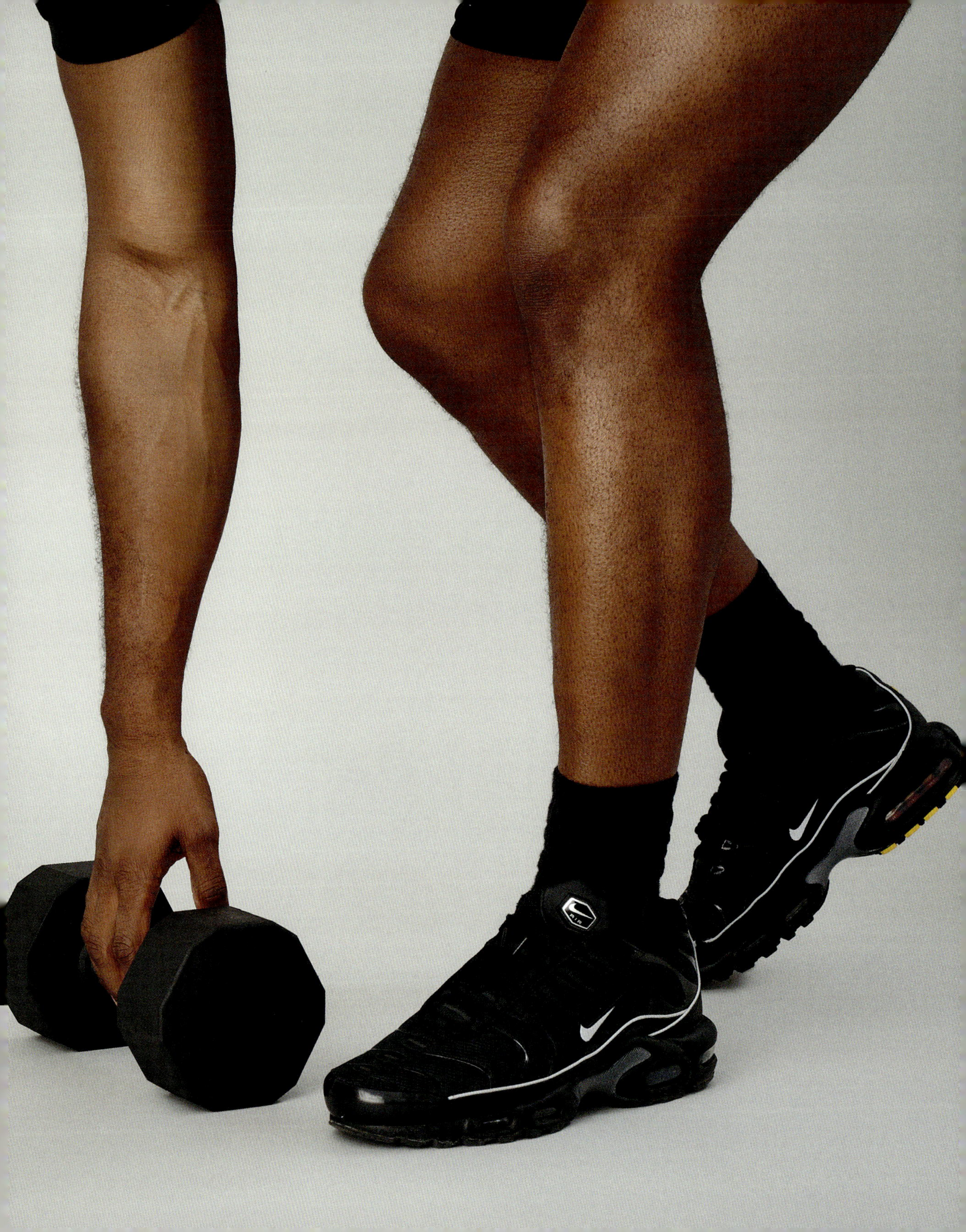

CHAPTER 2

Your Fitness Foundation

Building Your Routine

There's a saying that if you fail to plan, then you plan to fail. Let's spin it more positively: A good workout routine is one you tailor to remain consistent and focus on the results you want.

In this program, we'll focus on basic fundamental exercises that work your body primarily through compound exercise, which works several muscle groups at once. This approach saves a lot of time and energy, plus it's applicable for developing functional strength and longevity. This is because these exercises develop more than just strength—they also increase stability, mobility, and coordination.

Some of the most common target approaches are pulling exercises, pushing exercises, and squatting exercises.

- **Pulling exercises** work your muscles by pulling your hands toward your torso against resistance to work the muscles in your back and biceps, like when doing a row or pulling down on resistance bands.

- **Pushing exercises** involve pushing your hands away from your torso against resistance, like when doing a push-up or an overhead press, such as pressing dumbbells up overhead.

- **Squatting exercises** work your entire lower body with exercises like squats, lunges (stepping forward as you squat), and step-ups.

To round out your program, we'll also include additional techniques to focus on areas such as the abdominals, hips, and arms.

Most of these workouts involve working the entire body at once in a very efficient manner to create a holistic approach to strength training. Other plans will rotate through our target areas to add variety and ensure you place enough emphasis on each muscle group to prevent weaknesses and imbalances.

How to Structure Your Daily Workout

Structuring your daily workout doesn't need to be complicated. All you need to do is create the broad overview of your plan, then iron out the details as you zero in on your daily workouts. You can find formatted workout journals at a bookstore, but a simple note pad or the notes app on your phone will do fine to record your routine. I break it down into four steps.

STEP 1: PLAN YOUR WEEK

Start by planning your training for the week. In your calendar, write down which workouts you're going to do on which days of the week. I recommend practicing strength training two to three times a week, spending 20 to 40 minutes on a routine. Your routine doesn't need to last a certain amount of time to be effective, though—feel free to complete routines at your pace.

If you participate in other physical activities, such as organized sports, running, or hiking, plan your strength workouts around them. Ideally, you'll plan your workouts on days you're not doing other activities. If this isn't possible, use your best judgment to determine which days will give you the most time and energy to dedicate to each activity.

SAMPLE SCHEDULE

SUN	MON	TUE	WED	THU	FRI	SAT
Rest	Workout #1	Rest	Workout #2	Rest	Workout #3	Rest

STEP 2: PLAN YOUR EXERCISES FOR EACH WORKOUT

Once you've chosen your workout days, plan the exercises you'll practice in each workout. This can be pretty basic. You may choose to spend one day focusing on upper body, a second day on lower body, and the third on core. Sample routines for each target region are listed in chapters 3, 4, and 5, respectively. If you prefer, mix it up and focus on all three in a single workout.

SAMPLE ROUTINE

WORKOUT #1	WORKOUT #2	WORKOUT #3
Rows	Dumbbell Rows	Band Rows
Push-ups	Dumbbell Press	Plank
Squats	Lunges	Hip Extensions

STEP 3: CEMENT THE FINE DETAILS

Once you've settled on the exercises for each workout, map out how you'll practice each exercise. These details can include how much resistance, how many reps, and how many sets you'll do.

SAMPLE SPECIFICATIONS

WORKOUT #1	WORKOUT #2	WORKOUT #3
Rows Suspension 3 × 12 reps	**Dumbbell Rows** 25#/hand 2 × 8 reps	**Band Rows** Black band 3 × 14 reps/arm
Push-ups On back of couch 2 × 10 reps	**Dumbbell Press** 30#/hand single arm 12/side	**Plank** Holding for 3 × 30s
Squats 4 × 15 reps	**Lunges** BW alternating for 3 × 20 reps	**Hip Extensions** Heels on couch 2 × 20 reps

STEP 4: PRACTICE, ASSESS, AND PLAN ADJUSTMENTS FOR NEXT TIME

This fourth step is the most crucial and one you'll continue using to inform your workouts along your strength-training journey.

This step entails practicing a workout, recording and assessing how you did, and then planning how you can improve or adjust what you did for your next workout. Focus on technical points like your range of motion, stability, speed, and control, and do your best to not let those qualities erode under fatigue. Paying attention to those qualities and how they change throughout the workout will improve your proficiency; taking a moment to mindfully assess and plan your next workout can help you make tremendous strides moving forward.

SAMPLE POST-WORKOUT ASSESSMENT

WORKOUT #1	WORKOUT #2	WORKOUT #3
Rows Suspension 3 × 12 reps *Keep elbows in closer to sides*	**Dumbbell Rows** 25#/hand 2 × 8 reps *More reps next time*	**Band Rows** Black band 3 × 14/arm *Move at a faster tempo*
Push-ups On back of couch 2 × 10 reps *More reps next time*	**Dumbbell Press** 30#/hand single arm 12/side *Move to 35# dumbbells next workout*	**Plank** Holding for 3 × 30s *Move at a faster tempo*
Squats 4 × 15 reps *Use more range of motion*	**Lunges** BW alternating for 3 × 20 reps *Keeps hands on hips for more balance*	**Hip Extensions** Heels on couch 2 × 20 reps *Keep glutes tight at bottom of each rep*

Even though this book provides workout routines to get you started, your best results will come from creating custom routines that work with your schedule and preferences. For example, if you prefer to train on weekdays, modify the workout schedule to give you weekends off. If you find working your lower body twice a week leaves you too tired for a weekly run, change it to once a week and focus on other areas. Do whatever you need to make it yours.

Making Progress

Hopefully, you can see how building and documenting your workout routine gives you structure for a disciplined workout plan that also allows you to plan and track your progress.

Writing down your plan, and detailing how you will (and did) perform each exercise, are essential for long-term progress. Many people assume that success will come if you simply show up and put in the work, but this is a myth. Vowing to "just show up and work hard" is the biggest reason many people fail. A successful workout plan will keep your mind focused on what you need to do to improve over time.

Possible adjustments

- Getting in a few more reps on the next workout

- Maintaining control through the set so you're not using too much momentum

- Maintaining strict form so you're not moving your body to make the exercise easier, like leaning back during a pull-down

- Using a full range of motion

You don't need to chase perfection or make big changes from one workout to the next. Instead of increasing weight, look for subtle changes you can make in form and body control to improve efficacy over time.

As you progress, don't forget that all exercises are adaptable to suit your needs. It's natural for the body to adapt rather quickly to training, especially in the first several months of a new program. This adaptation lays the foundation for the increased strength, mobility, and stability that will fortify your longevity. It's also why your program and exercises must continue to adapt—to keep pace with your increasing abilities.

Most of the time, this will mean adding resistance, or weight, to continue challenging your growing muscles. Sometimes, you may need to reduce the resistance to work on improving stability and mobility in an exercise. These are the kinds of things to look for, to ensure your workout program is in alignment with your personal abilities and helping you accomplish your goals.

Now, let's get started!

Keep in mind during exercise

- With dynamic techniques, use as much range of motion as possible to promote mobility.

- Exhale while you lift against resistance, and inhale as you return to starting position. In the case of isometric exercises (pages 54, 60), breathe in for 2 to 3 seconds, and exhale for the same amount of time. Keep your breathing smooth and controlled. Avoid holding your breath.

- Maintain control. Avoid using momentum and excessive motion other than the working limbs being used.

- Keep the muscles you're working tense until you've finished the exercise. Maintaining some tension in the working muscles makes the exercise more effective and avoids stress in the joints.

SUN	MON	TUE	WED	THU	FRI	SAT

WORKOUT #1	WORKOUT #2	WORKOUT #3

CHAPTER 3

Upper Body

Though tempting, a common mistake with upper body exercises is to focus attention on the "mirror muscles"—that is, the muscles on the front of the body, including the muscles in the chest, biceps, and the front of the shoulders. These muscles are beneficial, but it's the muscles you *don't* see, on the back of the torso, that are far more important. In fact, the muscles in the back of your shoulders and upper back, as well as your lats and the muscles that run along your spine, play a vital role in maintaining healthy posture, helping your body withstand stress and avoid chronic back pain.

Unfortunately, these posterior muscles are the very muscles that weaken and contribute to the issues that threaten longevity. Much of this weakness is the by-product of our modern sedentary habits of sitting for hours at a time. Hunching over a portable screen has made these weaknesses more pronounced, affecting even young adults and teens.

Sedentary habits aren't the only culprit behind weak back muscles. Many seasoned athletes and hardcore fitness enthusiasts also suffer from having a weak back body. Prolonged training in a specialized sport or training discipline often leads to imbalances and hidden weaknesses due to a lack of holistic strength training. These imbalances compromise long-term health and, ultimately, longevity.

Back weakness isn't the only back issue that can compromise long-term health and resilience. The erosion of shoulder stability and mobility will also make anyone more fragile and injury-prone.

The exercises in these four upper-body routines are all designed to strengthen your entire back, while also developing mobility and stability for more resilient shoulders. These routines have been designed to place as little stress on your shoulder joints as possible while maintaining the efficacy that will build holistic strength throughout your back body.

ROUTINE #1

BAND PULL-APARTS

2 sets of 12–20 reps

ISOMETRIC CHEST PRESS

2 holds for 15 seconds each

WALL SNOW ANGELS

2 sets of 6–8 reps

SINGLE-BAND ROWS

3 sets of 6–10 reps each arm

STANDING DUMBBELL PRESS

3 sets of 8–12 reps each arm

Band Pull-Aparts

EQUIPMENT: Light resistance band
2 SETS OF 12–20 REPS

Starting position
Standing upright, hold your arms out straight at about eye level, holding the band with your hands about 2 feet apart.

The movement
Pull your hands apart to stretch the band while clenching your shoulders down and back and pressing your chest forward. Drop your hands slightly so the band touches the top of your chest.

Tip: Keep your arms tight to avoid bending your elbows. This way, your shoulders and upper back do most of the work.

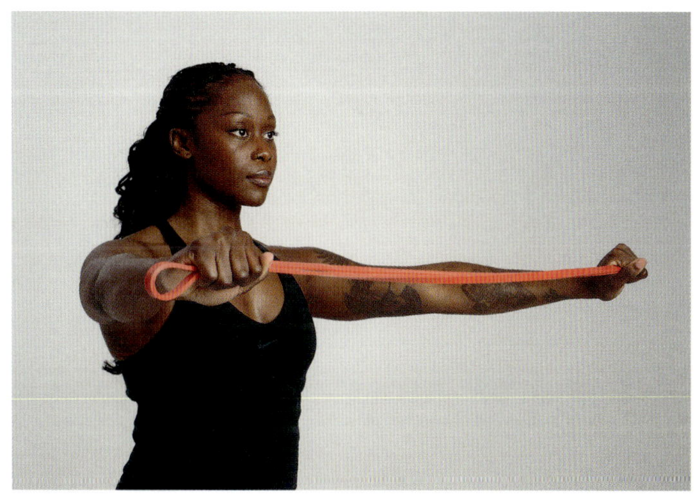

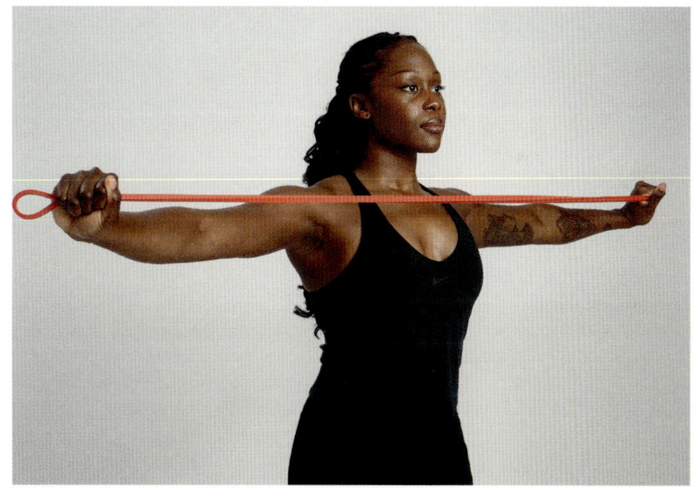

Isometric Chest Press

EQUIPMENT: None

2 HOLDS FOR 15 SECONDS EACH

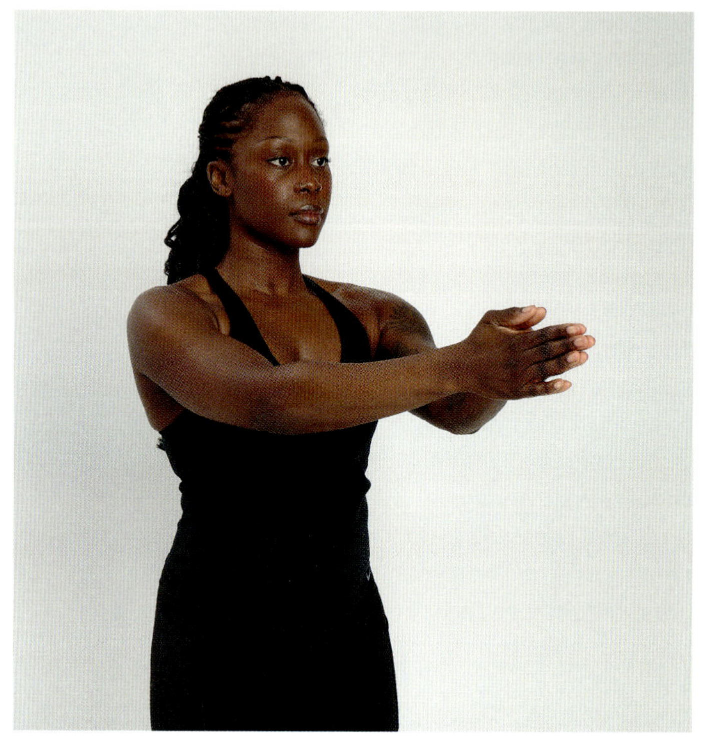

Starting position
Stand or sit upright with slightly bent arms outstretched at chest level, palms together and thumbs touching.

The movement
Take a deep breath, then exhale while forcefully pushing your palms together. Continue to press until you have exhausted all of your breath. Release when you breathe in.

Tip: Keep your elbows bent and low. Avoid hunching up your shoulders, which will make your elbows point out slightly to the side.

Wall Snow Angels

EQUIPMENT: Wall

2 SETS OF 6–8 REPS

Starting position

Stand with your back resting against the wall and your heels about 3 inches away from the base. Place the back of your hands against the wall with palms facing forward.

The movement

Slowly slide your arms out and upward against the wall like you're making a snow angel. Return by sliding your arms down to your sides.

Tip: Breathe smoothly through the motion, and don't force your range of motion; simply feel your shoulders working and the stretch in your back.

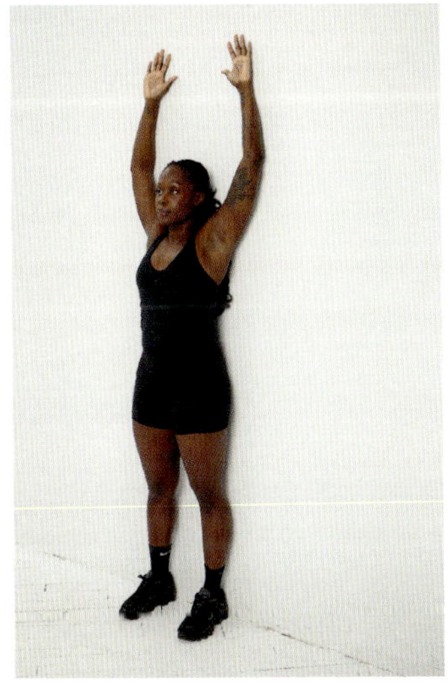

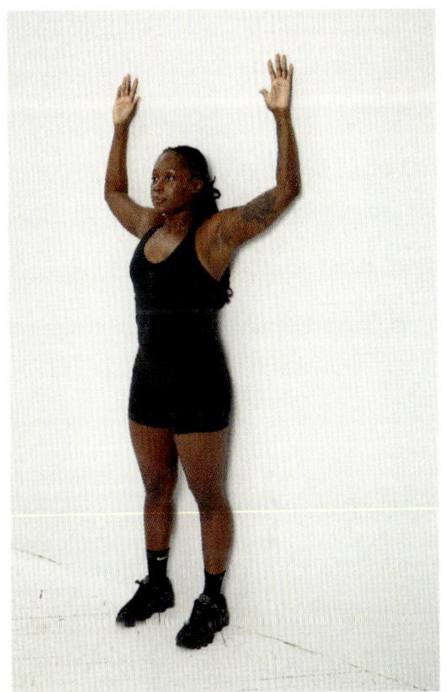

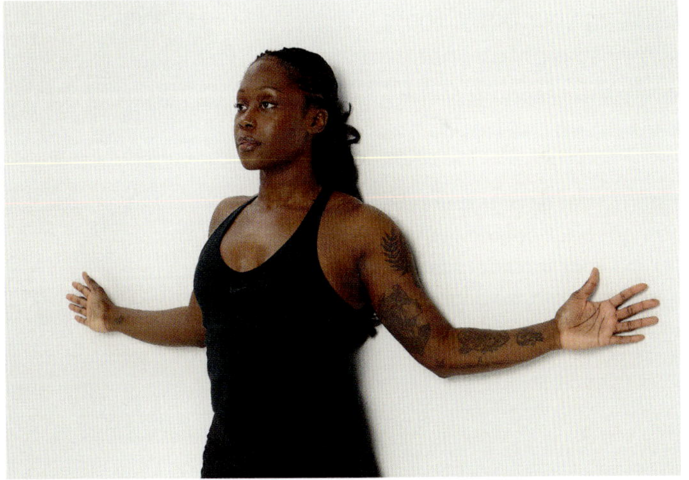

Single-Band Rows

EQUIPMENT: Moderate or heavy resistance band anchored to a sturdy support or door anchor

3 SETS OF 6–10 REPS EACH ARM

Starting position

Stand holding the band at chest level with one hand. Stand back far enough to get some stretch in the band. Step the opposite foot forward for support.

The movement

Pull the band back, keeping your arm close to your body, until your hand is at your lower chest without twisting your body. Then, slowly straighten your arm while maintaining some tension on the band.

Tip: Think of driving your elbow straight back behind you while pulling your shoulder blade down to maximize engagement of your back muscles.

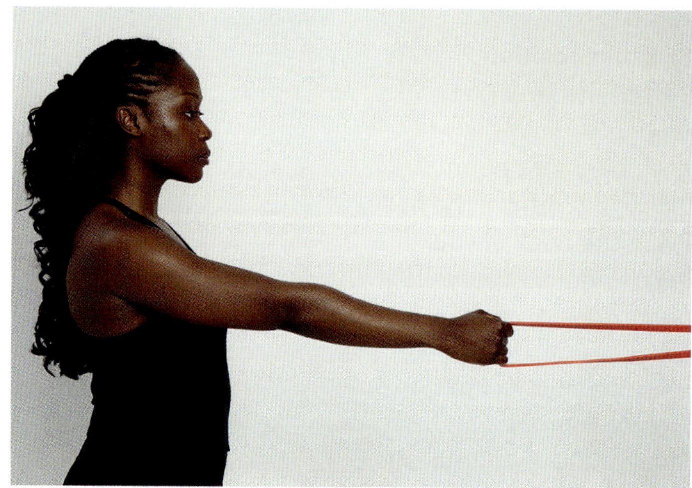

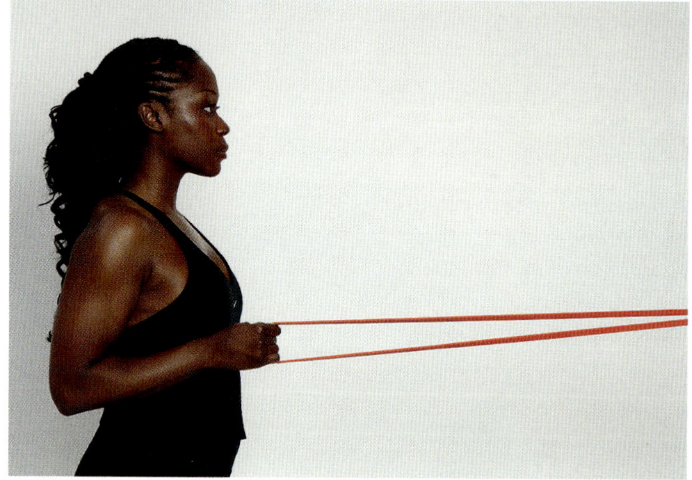

Standing Dumbbell Press

EQUIPMENT: Dumbbell

3 SETS OF 8–12 REPS EACH ARM

Starting position
Stand facing the anchor, with feet shoulder-width apart. Hold the dumbbell in one hand in front of your shoulder, palm facing you.

The movement
Press the dumbbell up overhead while rotating your arm so your palm is facing outward, away from you, at the top. Pause at the top, then slowly lower the weight in front of your shoulder.

Tip: Choose a dumbbell you can lift and lower with control. Keep your legs and core tight to prevent movement in your torso as you lift.

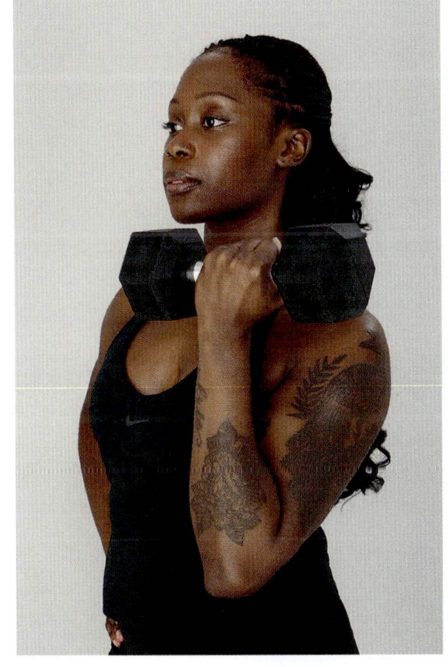

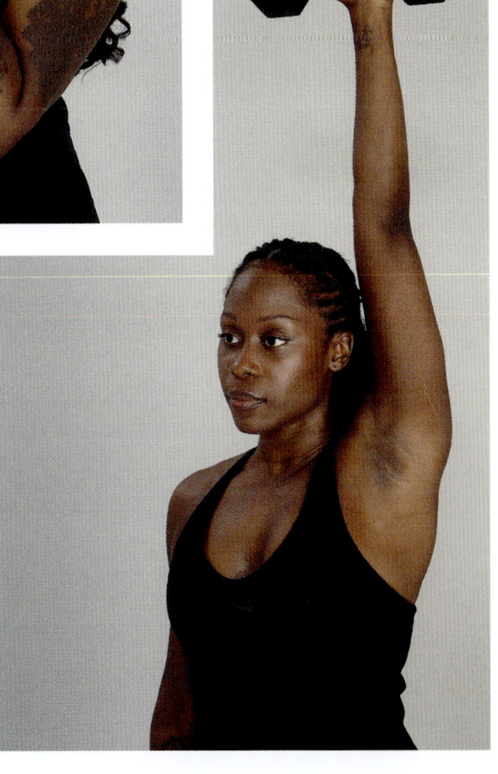

ROUTINE #2

STANDING SINGLE-BAND CHEST PRESS

2 sets of 12–15 reps each arm

ISOMETRIC BAND PULL-DOWN

3 holds for 15–20 seconds

BENT-OVER DUMBBELL ROW

2 sets of 8–12 reps

ALTERNATING SUSPENSION SHOULDER RAISES

2 sets of 14 reps

SUSPENSION BICEPS CURLS

2 sets of 12 reps

Standing Single-Band Chest Press

EQUIPMENT: Medium or heavy resistance band anchored to a sturdy support or door anchor

2 SETS OF 12–15 REPS EACH ARM

Starting position

Stand facing away from the anchor, holding the band with your elbow bent and the band resting outside your arm. Place the opposite leg in front for stability.

The movement

Press your arm forward and upward so the band rolls over the top of your shoulder. Return the hand to your side, allowing the band to return to the side of your shoulder.

Tip: Keep your legs and core braced to prevent movement in your upper body. It's fine to twist your body slightly as you press forward.

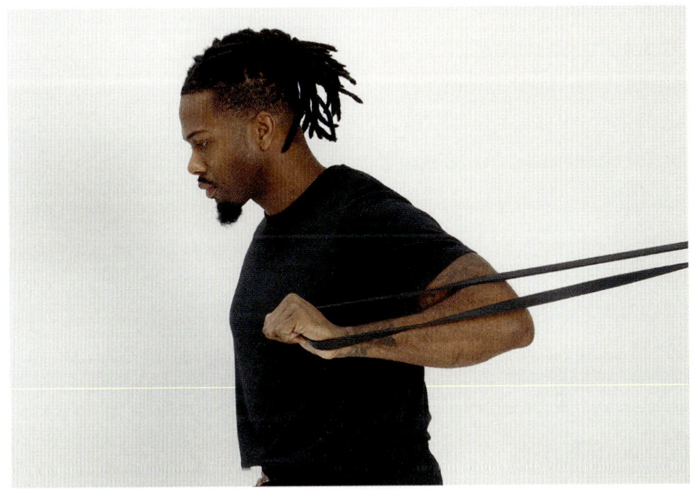

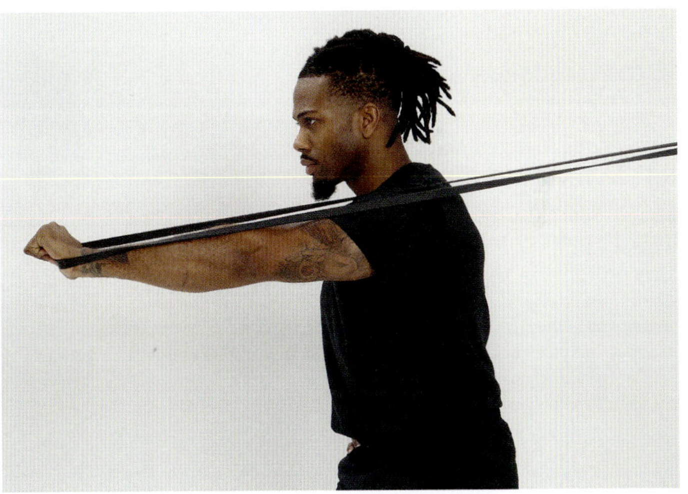

Isometric Band Pull-Down

EQUIPMENT: Moderate to heavy resistance band anchored to a sturdy support or door anchor

3 HOLDS FOR 15–20 SECONDS

Starting position

Sit on the floor facing the support or door, with legs outstretched and torso upright, holding the band anchored above you with both hands. Keep your torso upright.

The movement

Pull your hands down in front of your shoulders while driving your elbows tight to your sides. Hold for 15 to 20 seconds.

Tip: Try not to lean back to use your bodyweight to assist in the exercise. Bend your knees a bit, if that's more comfortable to stay upright.

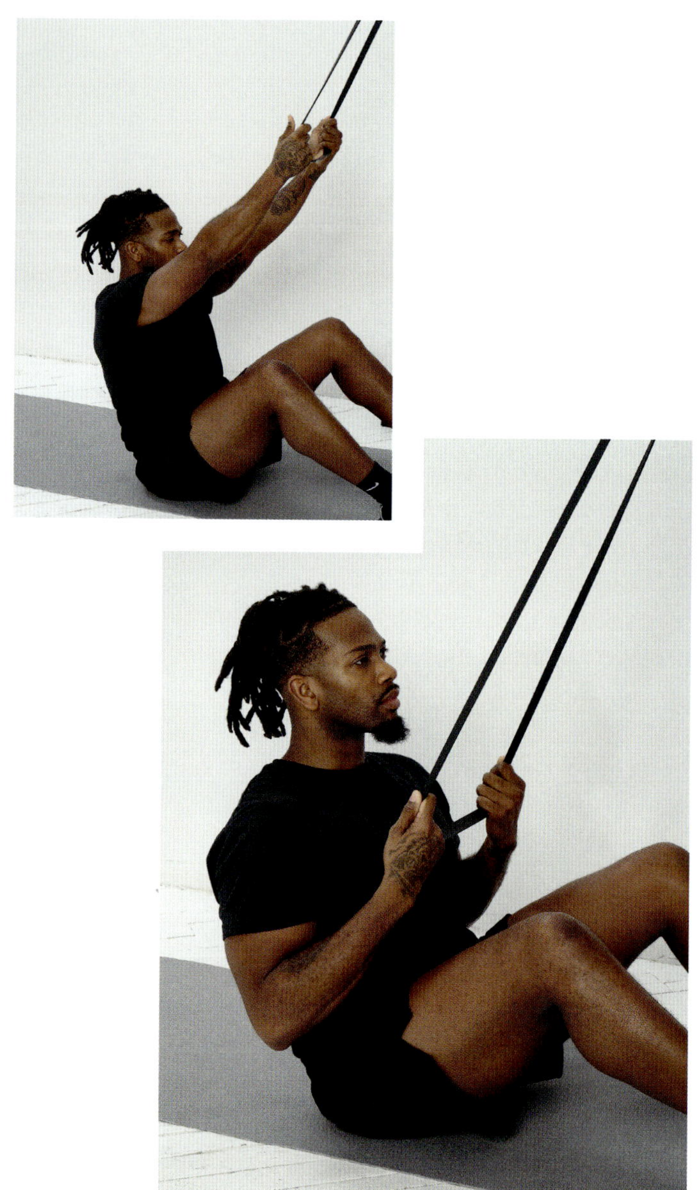

Bent-Over Dumbbell Row

EQUIPMENT: 2 moderate to heavy dumbbells

2 SETS OF 8–12 REPS

Starting position

Stand with knees bent slightly, and hinge at your hips to angle your torso forward about 45 degrees. With arms straight, hold the dumbbells directly over your feet.

The movement

Pull your elbows back to lift the dumbbells next to your torso while rotating your hands slightly so your palms face your lower ribs.

Tip: Maintain tension in your glutes (buttocks) and hamstrings (backs of thighs) while imagining squeezing your back toward your spine to provide stability in your lower back.

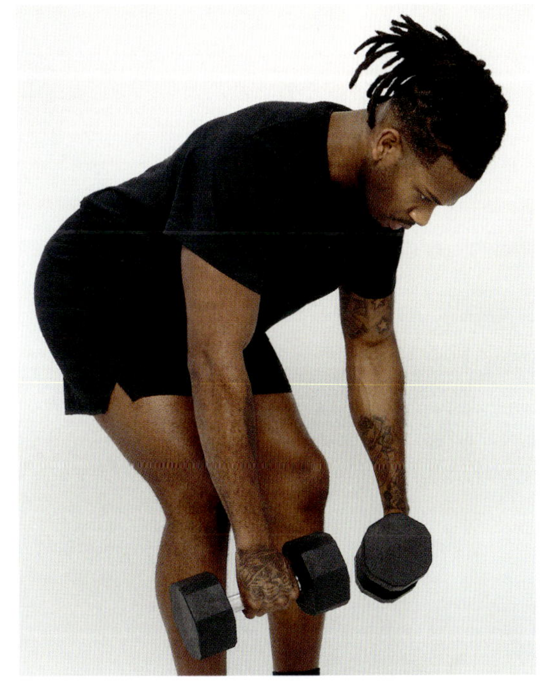

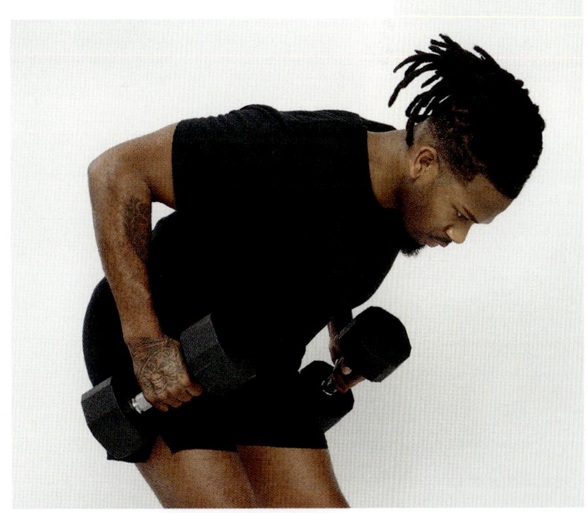

Alternating Suspension Shoulder Raises

EQUIPMENT: Suspension straps attached to an overhead support or door anchor

2 SETS OF 14 REPS

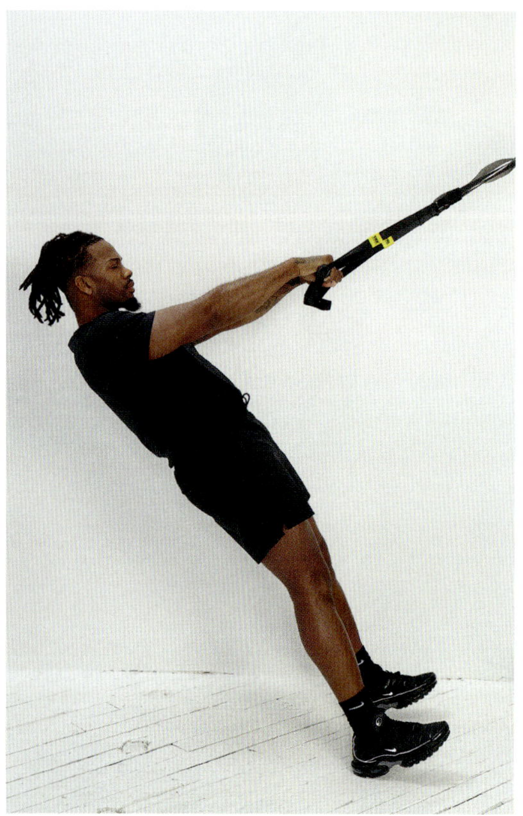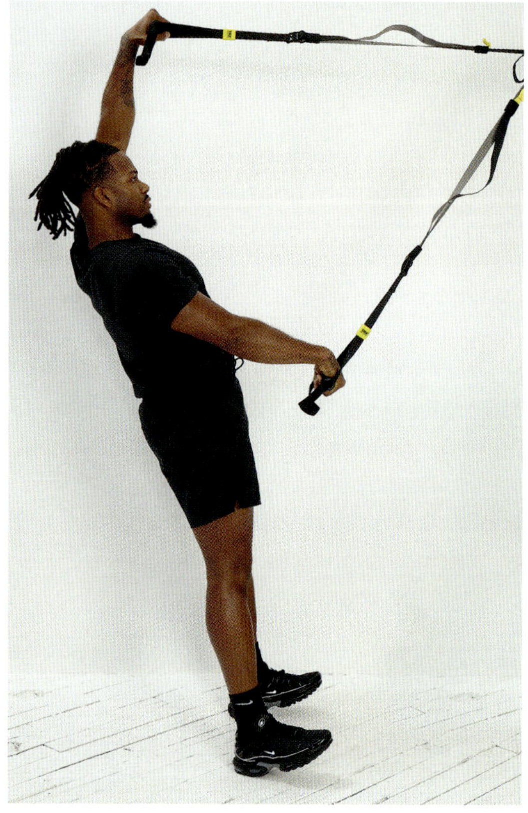

Starting position

Face the anchor point with your body leaning back slightly and arms straight out in front of you holding the straps.

Tip: Lift yourself only partway so you don't come completely upright, and let the straps sag, which removes the resistance.

The movement

Lift yourself almost fully upright by raising one arm straight up overhead while pulling the other arm straight down toward your hips. Pause slightly, then bring both hands together again in front of you. Repeat the motion on the opposite side.

Suspension Biceps Curls

EQUIPMENT: Suspension straps attached to an overhead support or door anchor

2 SETS OF 12 REPS

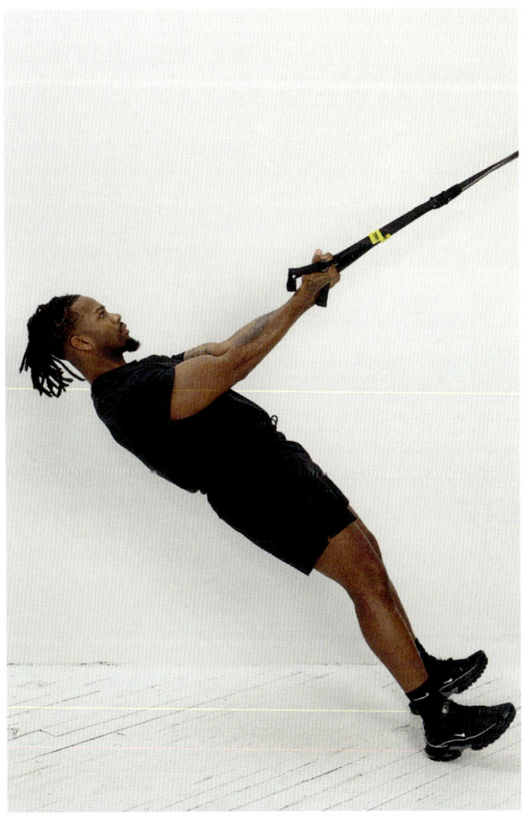

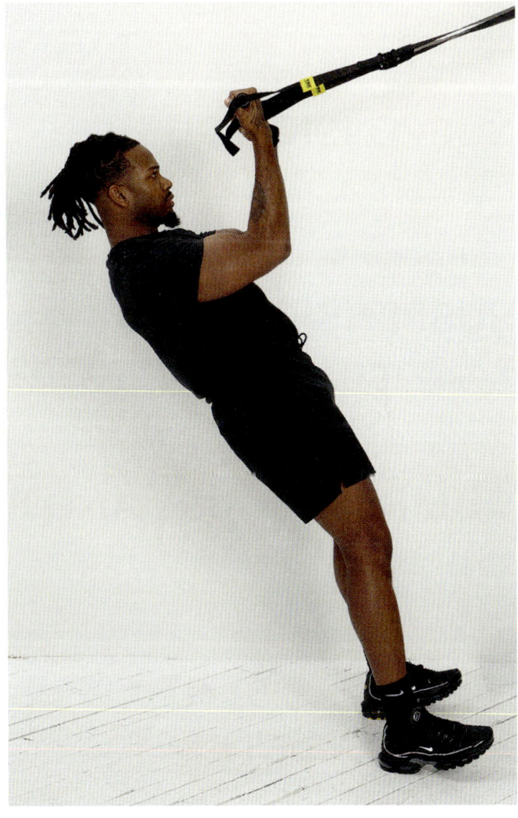

Starting position

Facing the anchor point, lean back with arms straight out in front of you, gripping the straps with palms facing upward and shoulders pulled back.

Tip: Think of "scooping" your hands upward as you lift yourself up. This will prevent your elbows from pulling down and back.

The movement

Pull your hands toward your face by bending your elbows to lift yourself up slightly, keeping your upper arms directly in front of you and turning your hands so the palms face you. Pause at the top, then lower yourself by straightening your arms with control.

ROUTINE #3

SUSPENSION PUSH-UP

3 sets of 8–12 reps

SUSPENSION ROWS

3 sets of 8–12 reps

DUMBBELL CURL AND PRESS

2 sets of 10–12 reps

DUMBBELL BENT-OVER STRAIGHT-ARM LAT PULL

2 sets of 10–12 reps

STANDING LATERAL-TO-FRONT DUMBBELL RAISE

2 sets of 6 reps

Suspension Push-Up

EQUIPMENT: Suspension straps attached to an overhead support or door anchor

3 SETS OF 8–12 REPS

Starting position

Face away from the anchor point with your weight on the balls of your feet and your hands out in front of you holding the straps, with the straps over your shoulders.

The movement

Bend your elbows, and lean forward between your hands, allowing the straps to move to the side of your shoulders. Pause at the bottom of the lean, then press your arms forward to push you back to starting position.

Tip: To maintain core strength and stability, keep your body straight, and don't allow your hips to sag forward.

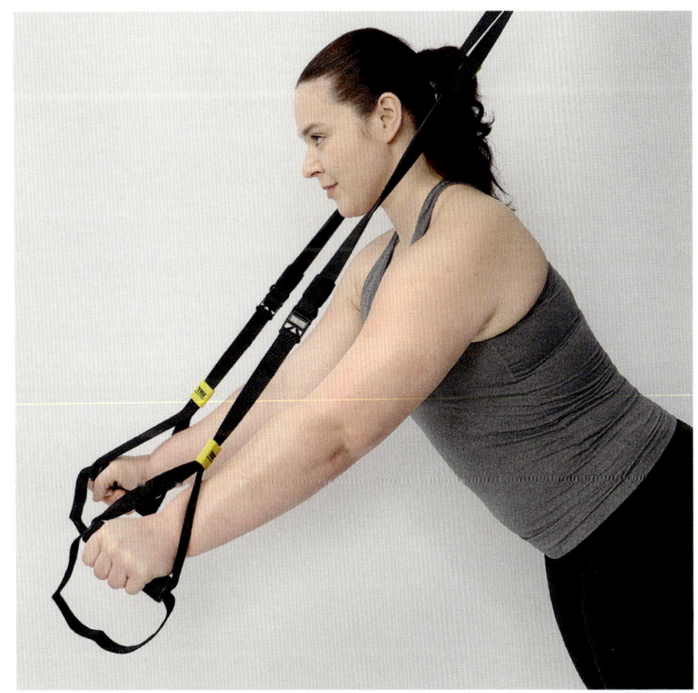

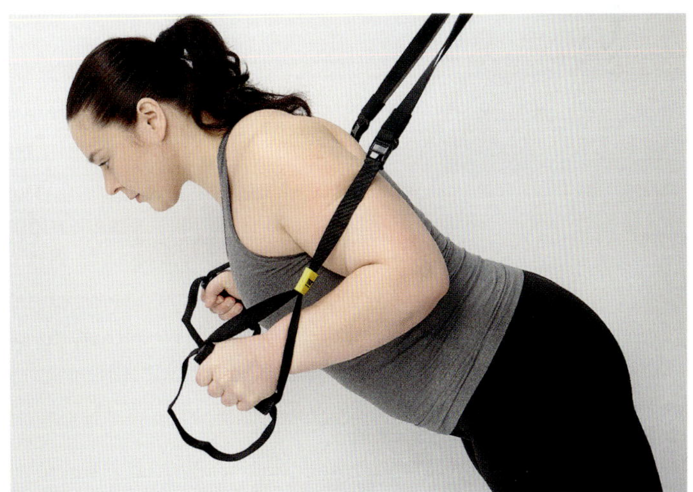

Suspension Rows

EQUIPMENT: Suspension straps attached to an overhead support or door anchor

3 SETS OF 8–12 REPS

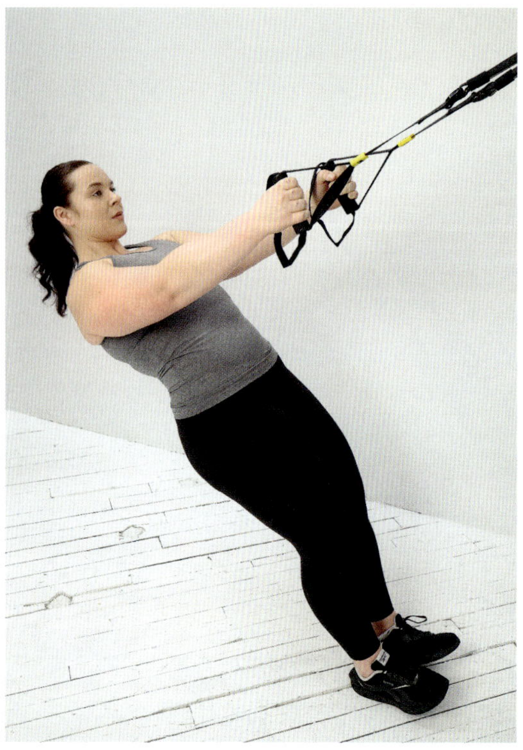

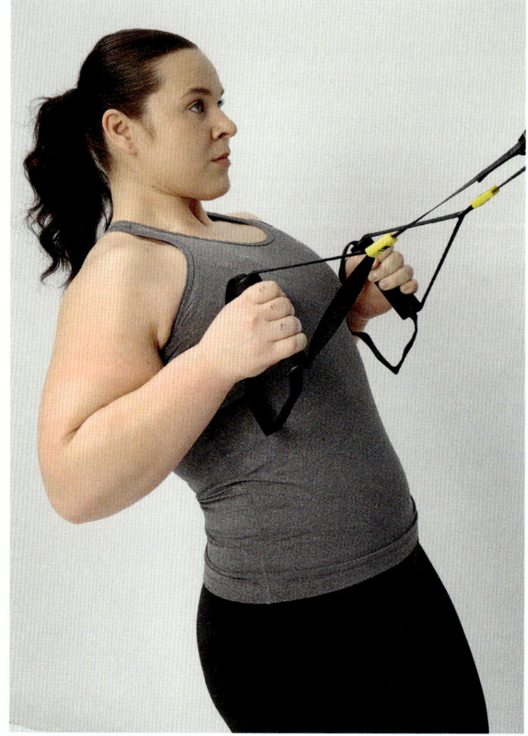

Starting position

Set the handles of the suspension straps at about waist height, and lean back with your arms straight, facing toward the anchor point. Knees can be straight or bent for traction.

Tip: Keep your wrists straight throughout the exercise, and activate your glutes to avoid driving your hips up for assistance.

The movement

Pull your torso up toward your hands by driving your elbows straight back behind you, keeping your hands close to your sides. Pull until your hands are at your lower chest, pause, and lower yourself slowly to starting position.

Dumbbell Curl and Press

EQUIPMENT: 2 light to moderate dumbbells

2 SETS OF 10–12 REPS

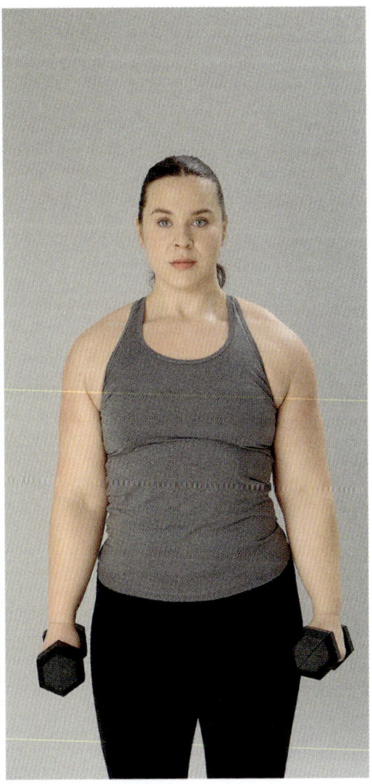 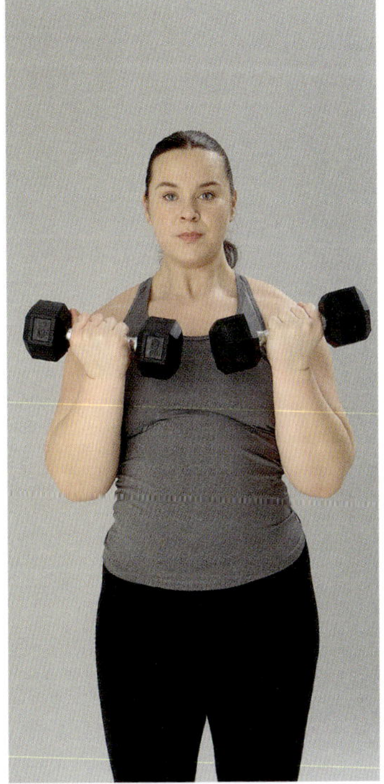 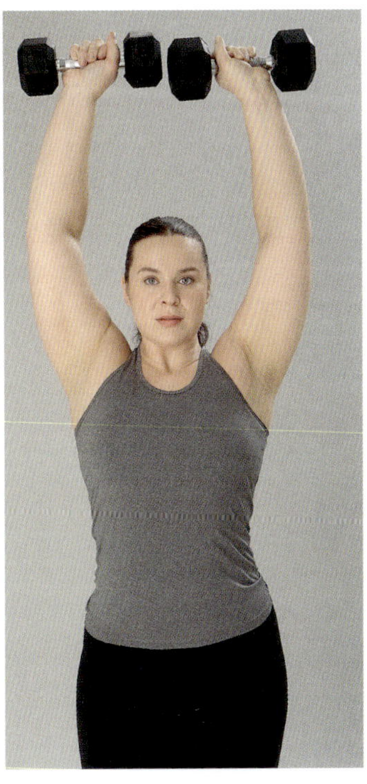

Starting position

Stand with feet shoulder-width apart, holding the dumbbells down by your sides.

Tip: Keep your shoulders back and abs tight to avoid swinging the weights forward at the bottom of each rep. If you can't help swinging, switch to lighter weights.

The movement

Lift the dumbbells up in front of you, bending at your elbows. Rotate your hands so your palms face your shoulders. Next, press both dumbbells up while rotating your hands until your arms are straight above your head, palms facing forward. Reverse the motion by lowering your hands to your shoulders and then down to your sides.

Dumbbell Bent-Over Straight-Arm Lat Pull

EQUIPMENT: 2 light dumbbells

2 SETS OF 10–12 REPS

Starting position

Stand and hinge at your hips to angle your torso forward about 45 degrees. With arms straight, hold the dumbbells directly over your feet.

The movement

Keeping your arms straight and gaze slightly forward, pull the weights back and upward toward your hips. Maintain a straight torso while pinching your shoulder blades together and down.

Tip: Move in a slow, smooth motion, pausing slightly at the top and bottom of each repetition to avoid swinging the dumbbells with momentum. If this is hard, try lighter dumbbells or even cans of soup.

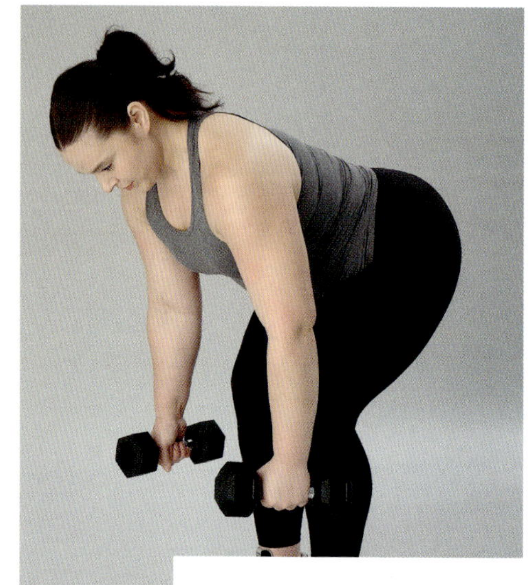

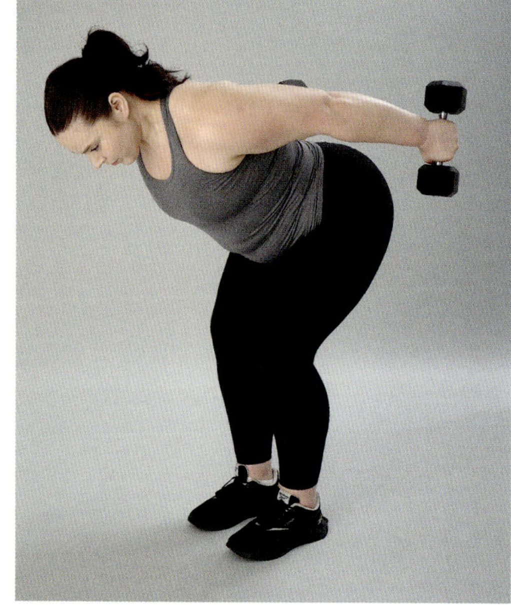

Standing Lateral-to-Front Dumbbell Raise

EQUIPMENT: 2 light dumbbells

2 SETS OF 6 REPS

Starting position

Stand with feet about 6 inches apart, holding the dumbbells down by your sides.

The movement

Lift your arms straight up and out to your sides until your hands are just below shoulder level. Bring your arms inward until they are straight out in front of you. Lower your hands down in front of you, keeping arms straight the whole time. Reverse the motion to return to starting position.

Tip: To make the exercise easier, keep your arms tight to avoid bending at the elbow. Try to reach the dumbbells out as far as you can to get as much range of motion as possible.

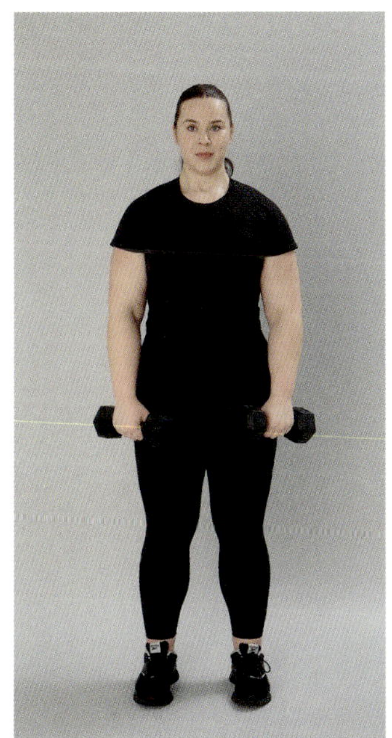
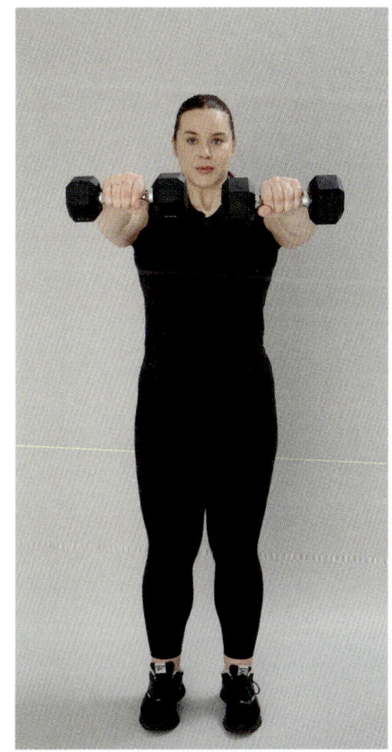
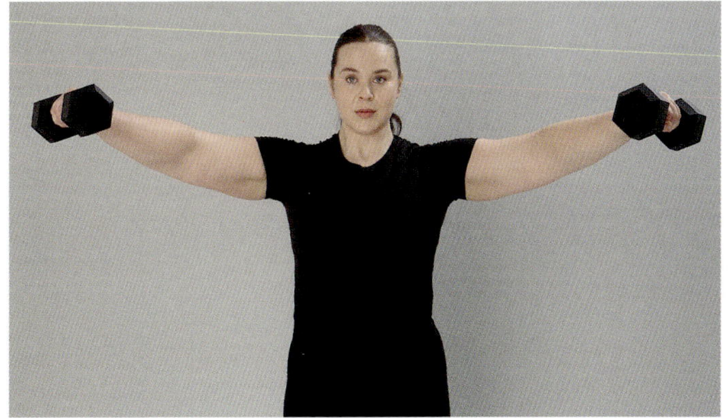

ROUTINE #4

BAND TRICEPS PRESS AND PULL-BACK

2 sets of 12–15 reps

BAND DOWNWARD CHEST PRESS

3 sets of 8–12 reps

BAND PULL-DOWN

3 sets of 8–12 reps

BAND UPRIGHT ROW

2 sets of 8–10 reps

STANDING SHOULDER ROLL

2 sets of 10 reps each direction

Band Triceps Press and Pull-Back

EQUIPMENT: Medium to heavy resistance band anchored to a sturdy support or door anchor

2 SETS OF 12–15 REPS

Starting position

Face the anchor point with arms bent and tucked in front of you, grasping the band in front of your chest. Lean forward slightly with your knees and hips flexed slightly.

The movement

Pull the band straight down by using your triceps (backs of upper arms) to straighten your arms. From there, pull your arms straight down and back behind you.

Tip: Experiment with choking up on the band to offer more resistance, or place your hands lower to make the exercise easier.

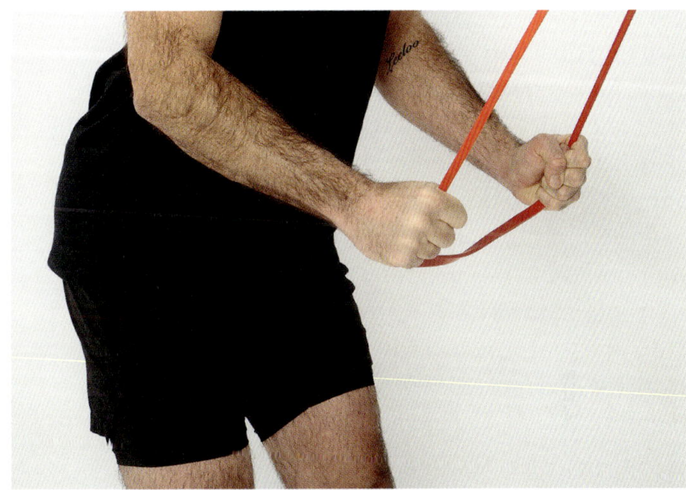

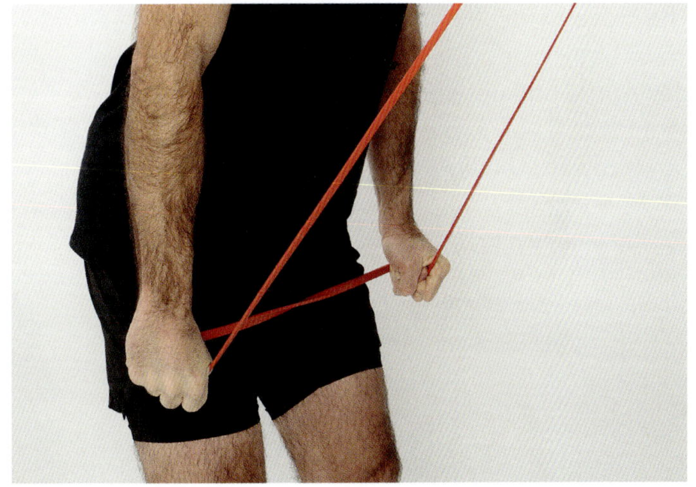

Band Downward Chest Press

EQUIPMENT: Medium to heavy resistance band anchored to an overhead support or door anchor

3 SETS OF 8–12 REPS

Starting position

Start facing away from the anchor point, 2 or 3 feet away from it, holding the bands with straight wrists. Bend your arms, and tuck your hands into your sides with your elbows back. Step one foot forward for stability, and lean forward slightly.

The movement

Press both hands downward and outward slightly, as if you're pushing down toward the floor.

Tip: Pay attention to your lower body to provide a strong and stable base while engaging your abs for support.

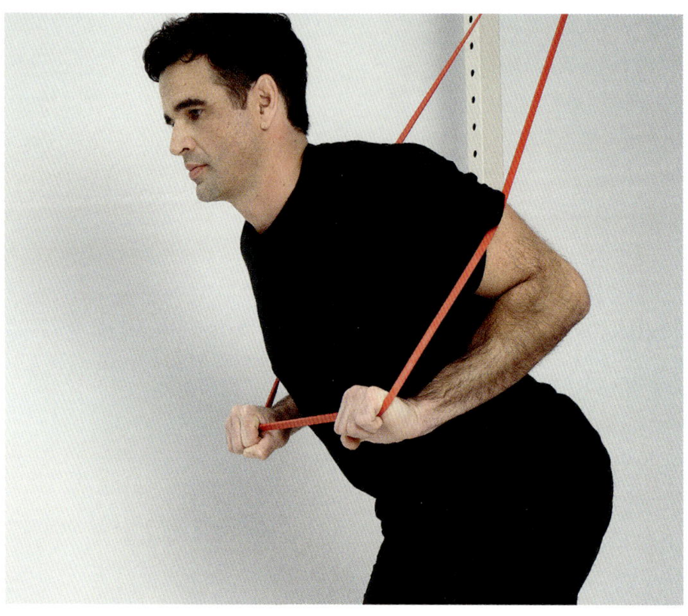

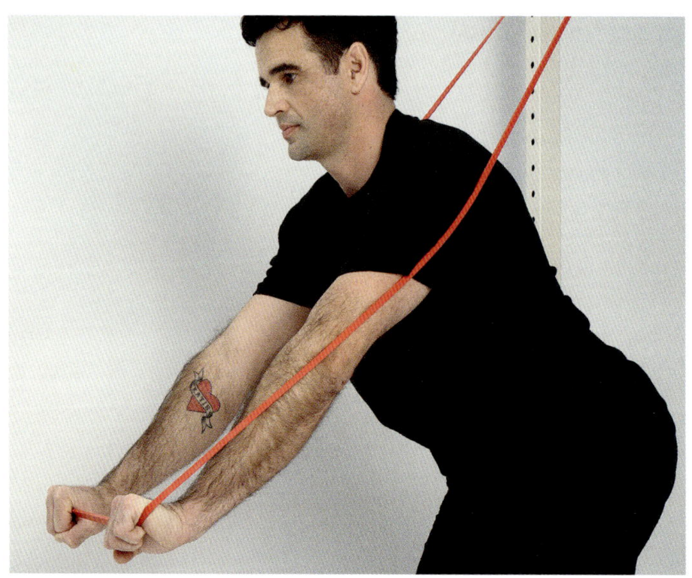

Band Pull-Down

EQUIPMENT: Medium to heavy resistance band anchored to a support or door anchor

3 SETS OF 8–12 REPS

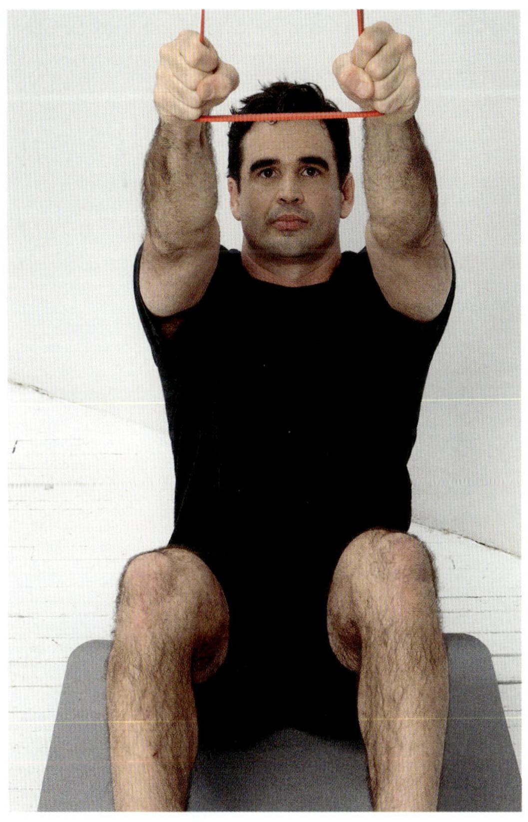 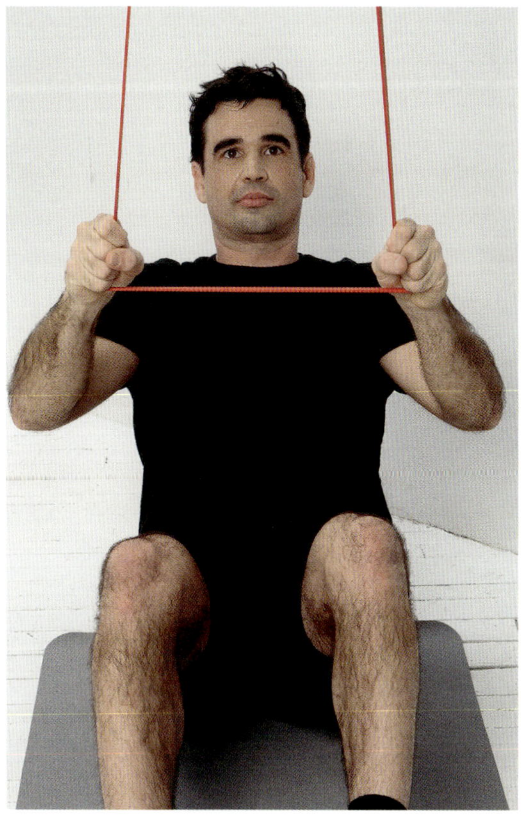

Starting position

Sit upright on the floor facing the anchor point with arms stretched up to grasp the band.

Tip: Rotate your hands as you pull so your palms face toward your upper chest in the bottom position. This can help engage your muscles while being gentler on your joints.

The movement

Pull your elbows down and into the sides of your torso, using the muscles in your back and biceps, while keeping your wrists straight.

Band Upright Row

EQUIPMENT: Light to medium resistance band

2 SETS OF 8–10 REPS

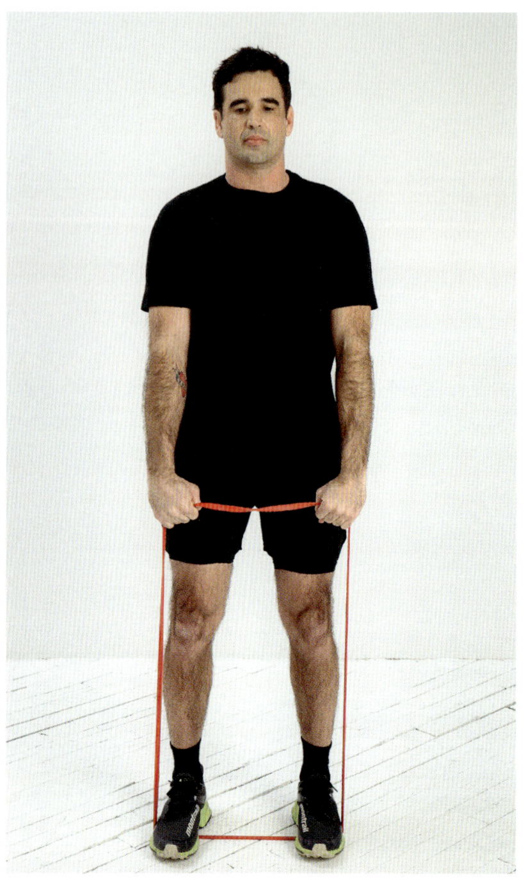

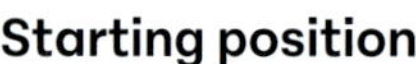

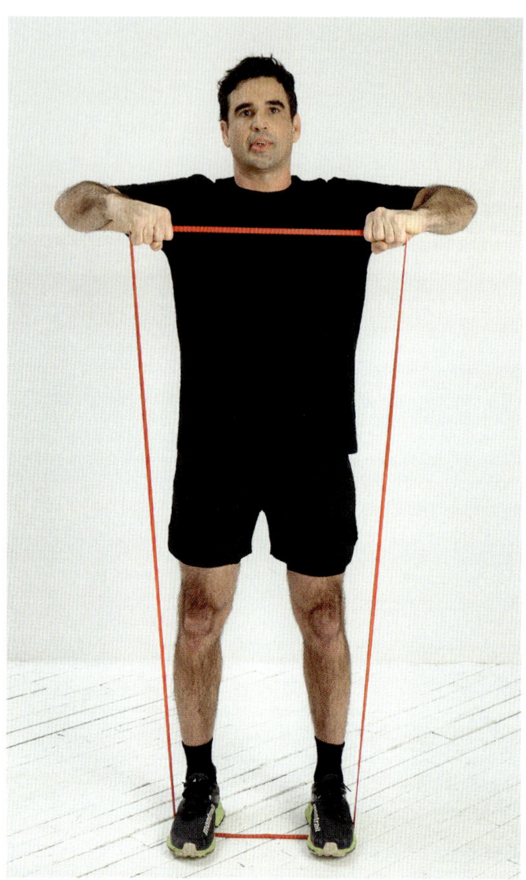

Starting position

Stand with the bottom of the band underneath your feet, about shoulder-width apart, secure under the arches of the feet so there's less chance of it slipping and snapping up. Hold on to the band with your arms straight down in front of you.

The movement

Pull your hands up toward your chest, lifting your elbows upward and out to the sides.

Tip: Lift your elbows in a smooth and controlled motion. Avoid using momentum to jerk your arms up. Keep your shoulder blades pinched behind you to support your shoulders.

Standing Shoulder Roll

EQUIPMENT: Medium to heavy resistance band or dumbbells (optional)

2 SETS OF 10 REPS EACH DIRECTION

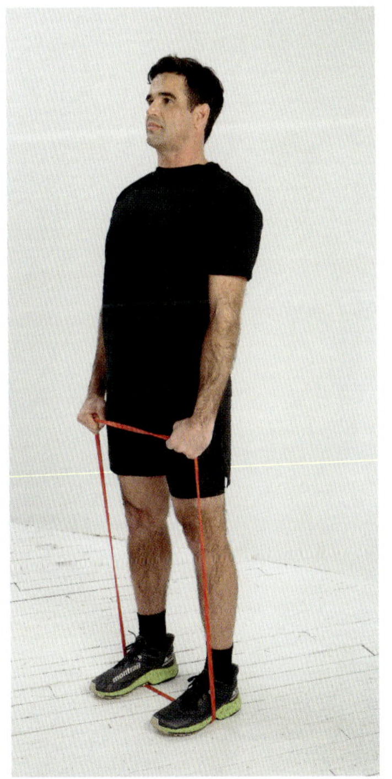 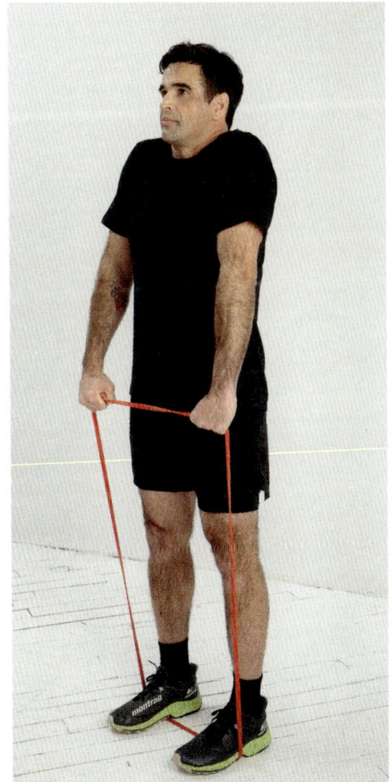 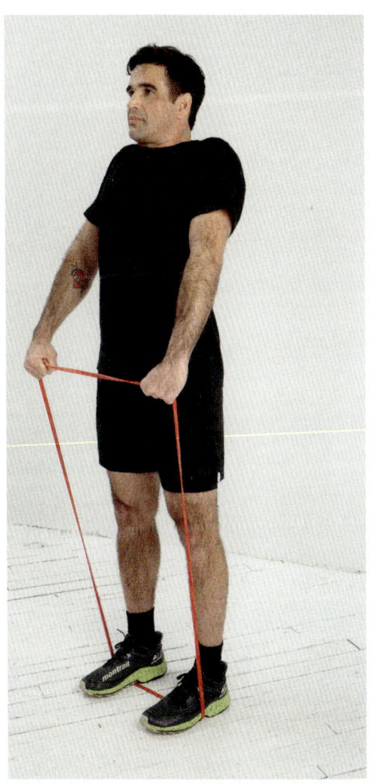

Starting position

Stand with feet about shoulder-width apart, with the bottom of the band secure under the arches of the feet so there's less chance of it slipping and snapping up. Hold on to the band with your arms down by your sides.

The movement

Roll your shoulders forward, up, and back in a circular motion using a wide range of motion. Think of spreading your shoulder blades apart when your shoulders are in front of you. In the top position, shrug your shoulders up toward your ears. Pinch your shoulders together when rolling back, and pull them downward at the bottom. Perform the same number of repetitions in each direction.

Tip: You can also do this exercise without any equipment as a stretching range of motion exercise.

CHAPTER 4

Lower Body

A strong and resilient body always starts from the ground up. This simple fact has been observed through the ages by athletes, martial artists, and even day laborers. It doesn't matter if you're a master of pull-ups and push-ups; when the legs get weak, the body as a whole becomes frail.

As with the upper body, lower-body strength alone isn't enough to ensure your legs will support a resilient body. Stability and mobility are also essential for your daily performance as well as longevity. Many gym goers use leg presses, hack squats, and other similar leg machines, which are great for building muscle and strength, but they don't address stability or mobility, especially in the hips. Combine these seated leg machines with our tendency to sit all day, and it's no wonder stability and mobility are in short supply these days.

It's easy to ignore the erosion of lower body stability and mobility, especially when our modern living can be so accommodating. It's especially easy to not notice a lack of functional strength when you're lifting on fancy weight machines. That is, until you slip on a slick floor or lift something heavy and something suddenly goes "POP!"

Sometimes the resulting issues aren't acute but rather build up into chronic issues. Conversely, a strong and stable lower body helps keep the whole body in proper alignment, including the hips, lumbar spine, shoulders, and neck. This may explain why many back and shoulder issues are caused by a lack of resilience in the lower body.

The exercises in this chapter have been carefully selected to develop strength, stability, *and* mobility. Each routine includes exercises that may emphasize strength, stability, or mobility, but requires all three elements of functional strength in a holistic approach to longevity.

ROUTINE #1

FRONT-TO-BACK SHIFTING LUNGES

2 sets of 8–10 reps each leg

CHAIR SQUATS

3 sets of 12–20 reps

WALKING WITH HIGH KNEES

20–30 reps or for distance

ROMANIAN DUMBBELL DEADLIFT

3 sets of 12 reps

WALL SIT

3 sets for 15–30 seconds each

Front-to-Back Shifting Lunges

EQUIPMENT: Exercise mat or folded towel for support, wall for support (optional)

2 SETS OF 8–10 REPS EACH LEG

Starting position

Step one foot forward, and bend both legs to crouch down into a low lunge position, so your back knee and toes rest on the floor and front shin is vertical with the foot directly under the knee.

The movement

Shift your weight forward onto the front leg and then back again.

Tip: Place feet shoulder-width apart for stability, and keep your weight pressed into the heel.

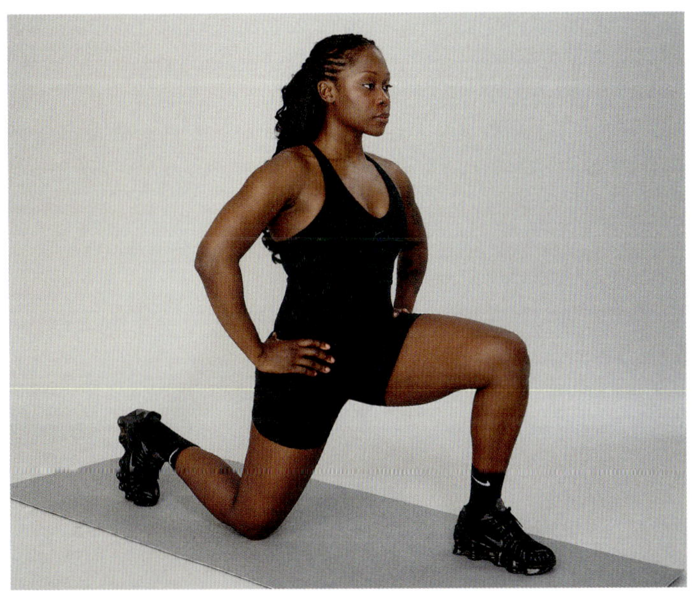

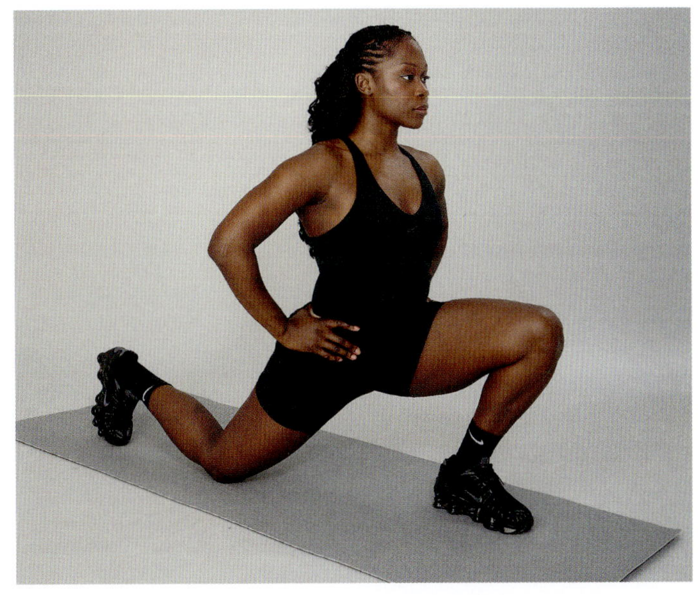

Chair Squats

EQUIPMENT: Sturdy chair

3 SETS OF 12–20 REPS

Starting position

Stand in front of the chair with your heels a couple of inches away. Hold the feet slightly wider than shoulder-width apart, toes pointed outward slightly, and hold your arms straight out in front of you, for balance.

The movement

Sit back with your hips while bending your knees over your toes, just like sitting back in a chair. Let your hips gently touch the chair before standing up again.

Tip: Try not to sit fully on the chair. Keep your muscles tense, and just "kiss" the chair with your hips, using control.

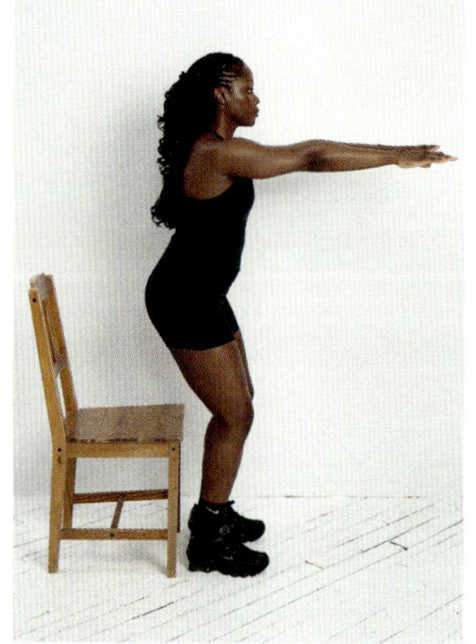

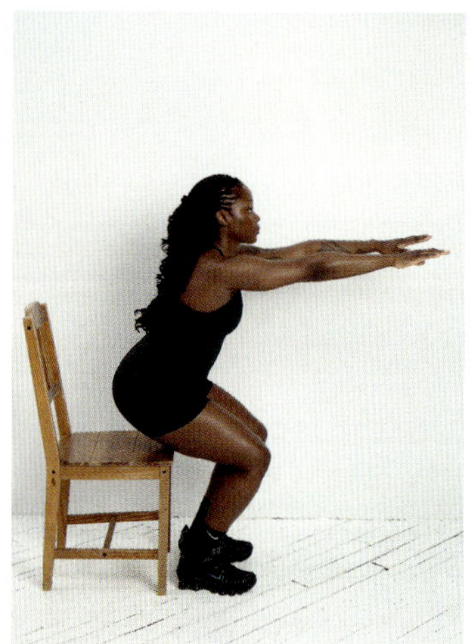

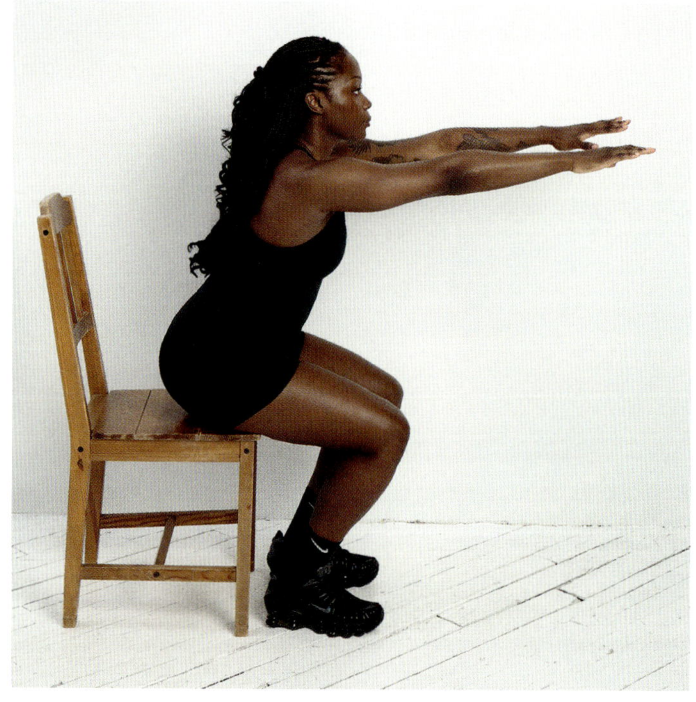

Walking with High Knees

EQUIPMENT: None

20–30 REPS OR FOR DISTANCE

Starting position
Stand with both legs strong, and step one leg forward slightly.

The movement
Start by standing on your stronger leg. Lift your knee as high as you can while bending your knee tightly, like you're trying to touch the back of your heel to your thigh, and pause. Set it down under control, and repeat on the other leg, alternating back and forth to complete the set.

Tip: Keep your standing leg and hip tense to improve stability and prevent leaning back with the upper body.

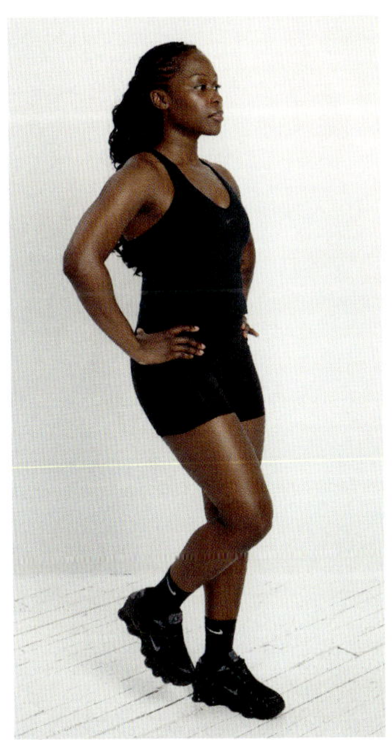
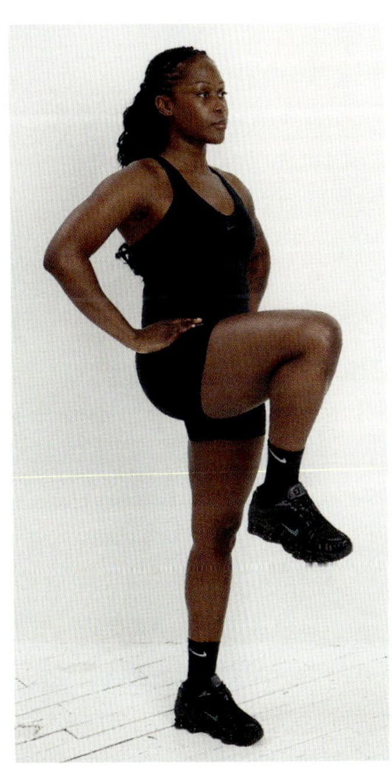

Romanian Dumbbell Deadlift

EQUIPMENT: 2 moderate to heavy dumbbells

3 SETS OF 12 REPS

Starting position

Stand with feet at least shoulder-width apart, holding the dumbbells down by your sides.

The movement

Hinge by pushing your hips back, and lean your torso forward while sliding the dumbbells down the front of your legs. Pause when you feel a light stretch in your hamstrings. Push your hips forward to reverse the motion, and rise to starting position.

Tip: Keep your shoulders pressed down and back to maintain a straight spine and stable lower back.

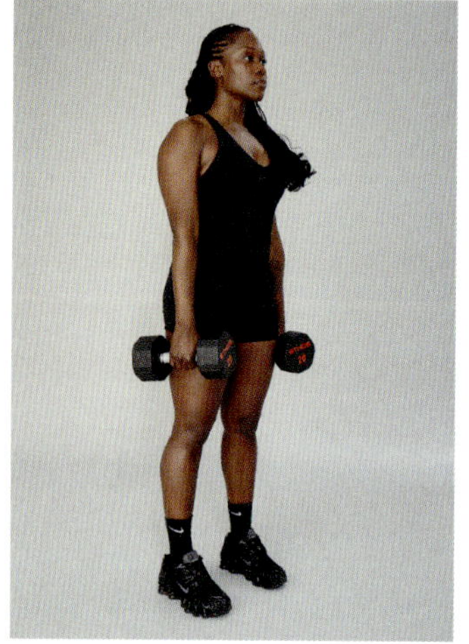
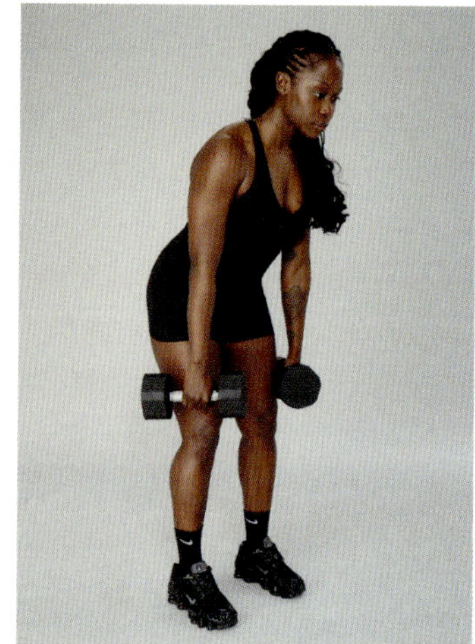
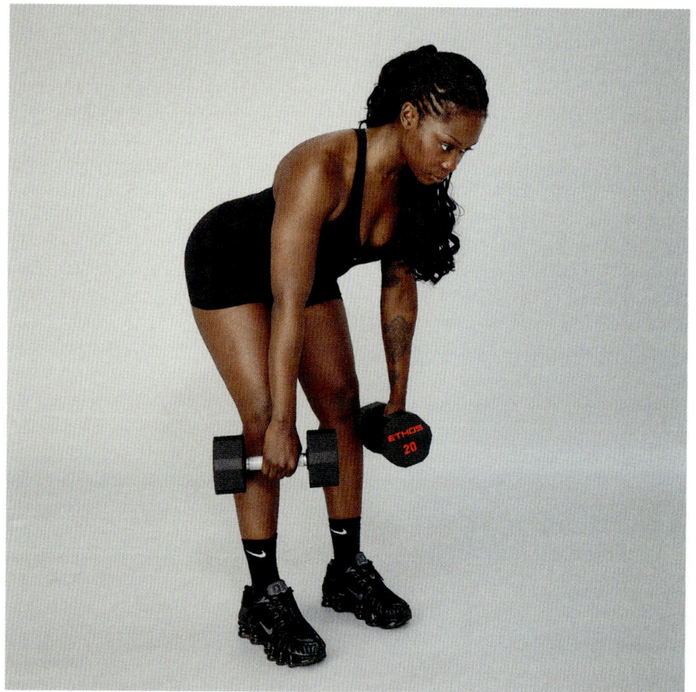

Wall Sit

EQUIPMENT: Sturdy wall, preferably with a smooth surface

3 SETS FOR 15–30 SECONDS EACH

Starting position

Stand about one step away from the wall, and lean forward slightly so your tailbone is touching the wall.

The movement

Slide your tailbone down the wall until your thighs are horizontal, and hold the position. Push your hands against the wall behind you to stand when finished.

Tip: Press into your heels to avoid stress in the knees.

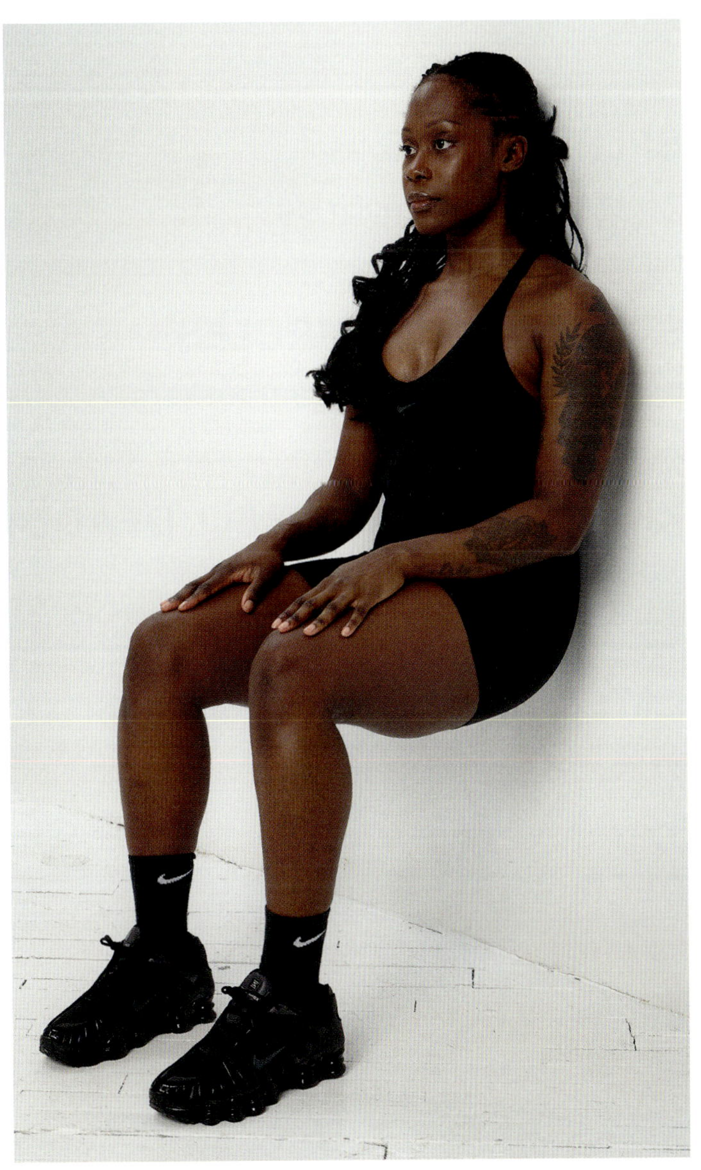

ROUTINE #2

SPLIT SQUATS

2 sets of 12–15 reps each leg

STANDING HIP CIRCLES

2 sets of 6–8 reps inward and outward

KICKSTAND DUMBBELL DEADLIFT

2 sets of 10 reps each leg

LATERAL SHIFTING SQUATS

2 sets of 8 reps

DEEP GOBLET SQUATS

2 sets of 6–8 reps

Split Squats

EQUIPMENT: 2 light to moderate dumbbells (optional)

2 SETS OF 12–15 REPS EACH LEG

Starting position

Place one foot a long stride in front of you with your feet shoulder-width apart. If using dumbbells, hold them down by your sides.

The movement

Bend your front knee over your toes to lower your hips closer to the back heel of your front leg. Pause with your back knee about 1 inch off the floor, and press up with the front leg.

Tip: Keep your weight on the heel of your front foot, and lean your torso forward slightly as you descend. Doing this helps with stability and puts less stress on the knees.

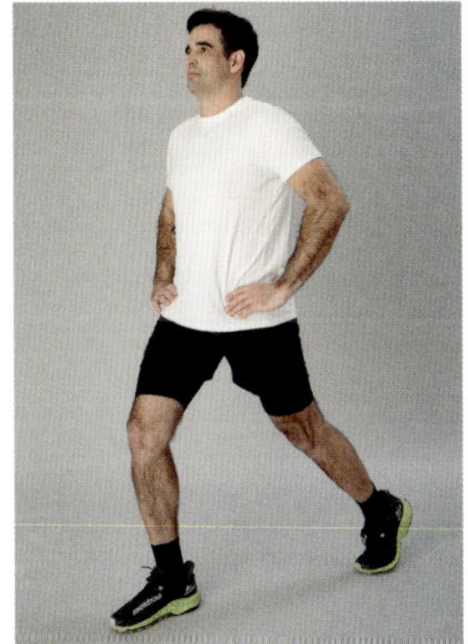
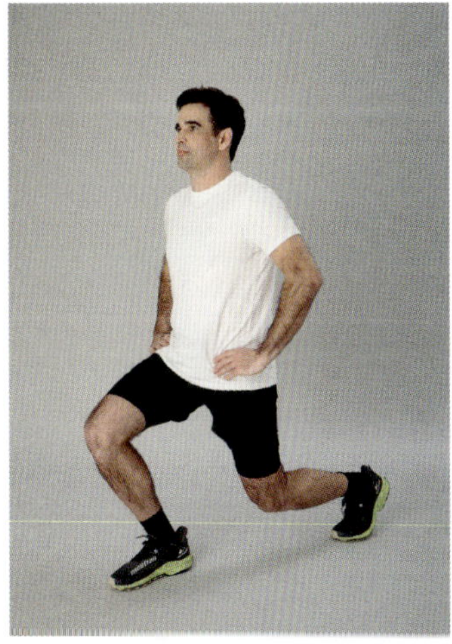
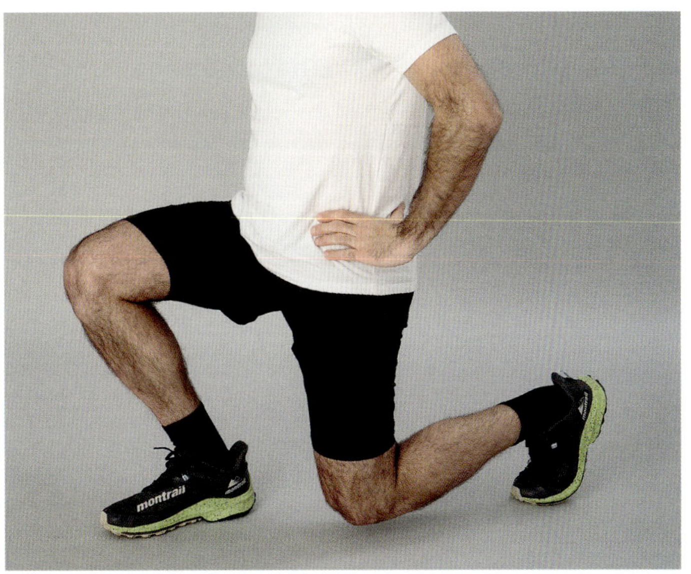

Standing Hip Circles

EQUIPMENT: Wall or sturdy chair for support (optional)

2 SETS OF 6–8 REPS INWARD AND OUTWARD

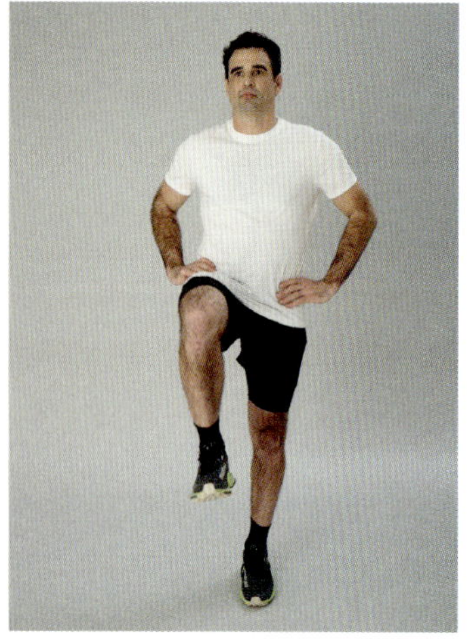 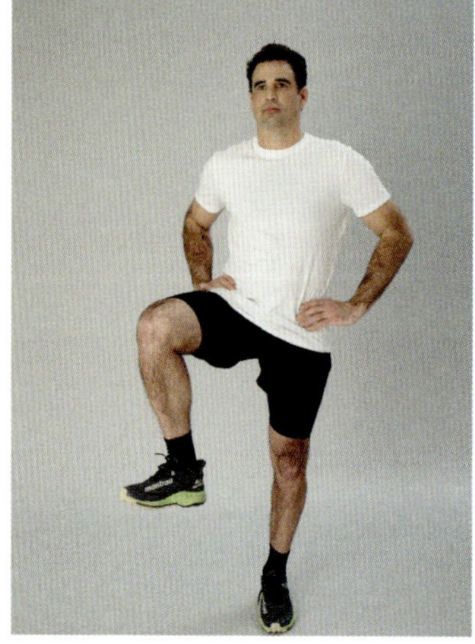 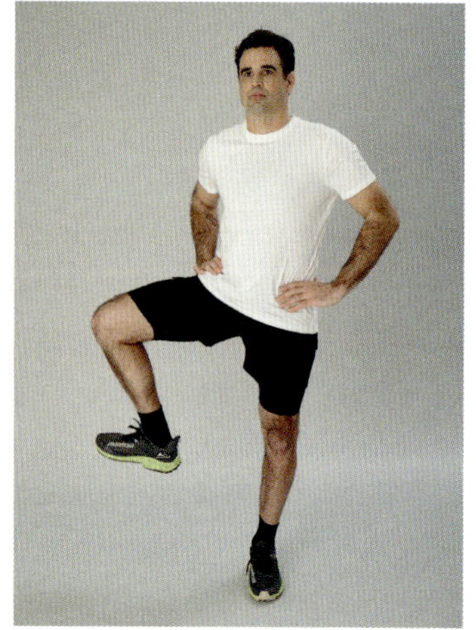

Starting position

Stand on one leg, and pick up the other knee in front of you as high as possible.

The movement

Rotate your upper leg outward to the side, down, in, and back up to draw a big circle with your knee. Perform the movement in a smooth motion with as much range as possible in both directions.

Tip: Keep the standing leg and hip tight to prevent twisting or moving the upper body as much as possible.

Kickstand Dumbbell Deadlift

EQUIPMENT: 2 light to moderate dumbbells

2 SETS OF 10 REPS EACH LEG

Starting position

Stand with both feet together, holding the dumbbells down by your sides. Bend one knee, placing that foot behind you slightly as a "kickstand," with toes touching the ground.

The movement

Hinge forward, pushing your hips back and sliding the dumbbells forward to slide down your front leg. Bend your front knee slightly to keep your shin vertical. Push your hips forward to stand up, bringing the dumbbells back up while keeping the shoulders pressed back and spine straight.

Tip: Place as little weight as possible on the rear foot so this exercise has as much of a single-leg deadlift as possible.

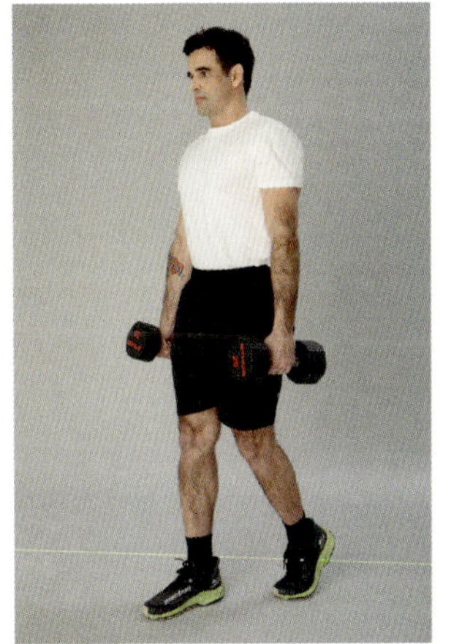

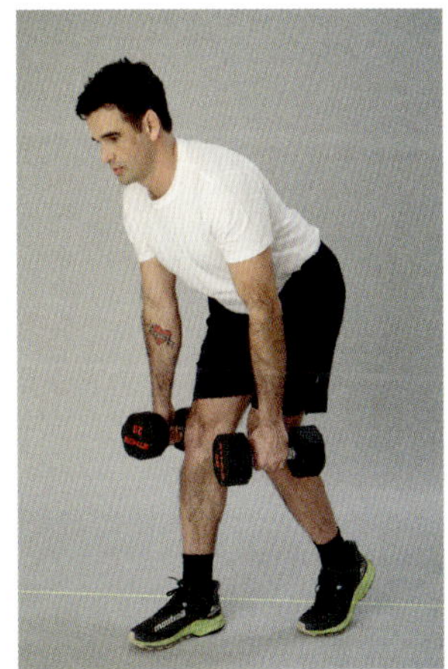

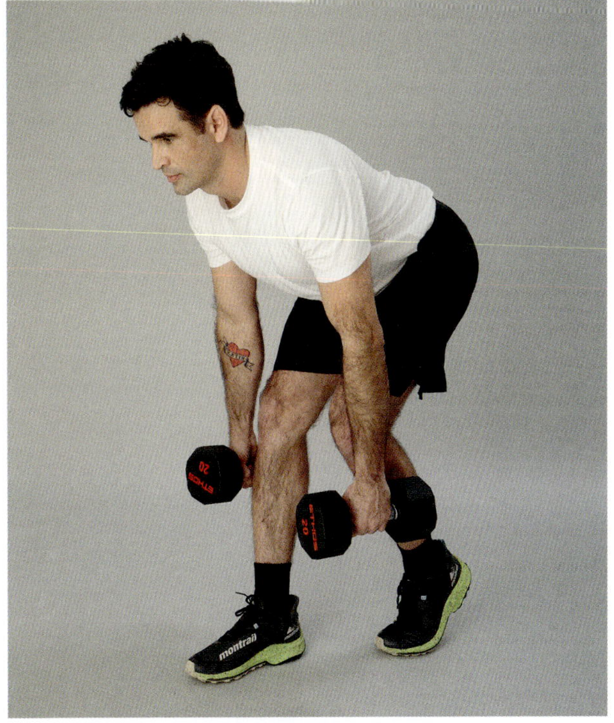

Lateral Shifting Squats

EQUIPMENT: None

2 SETS OF 8 REPS

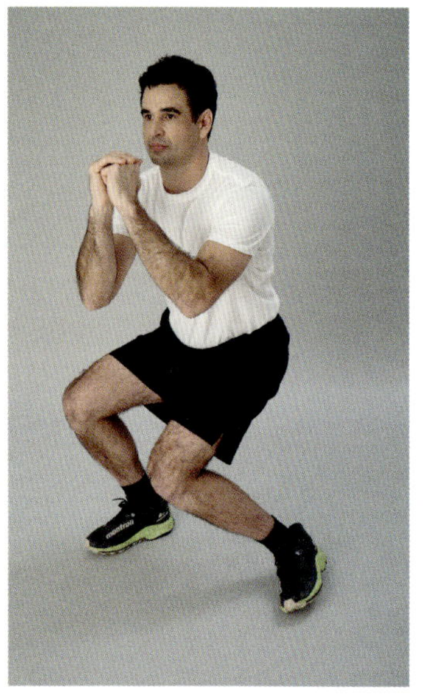 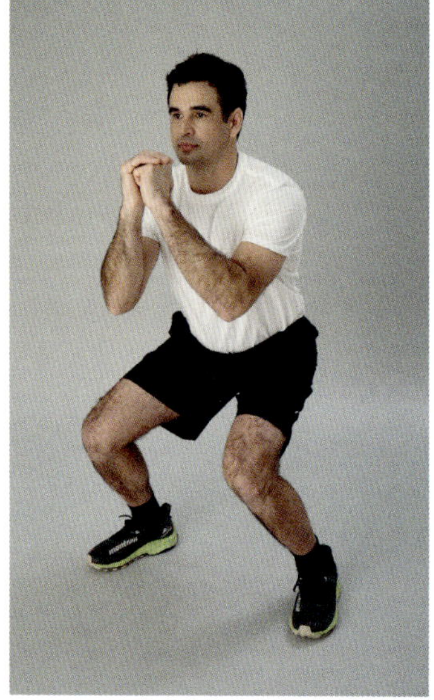 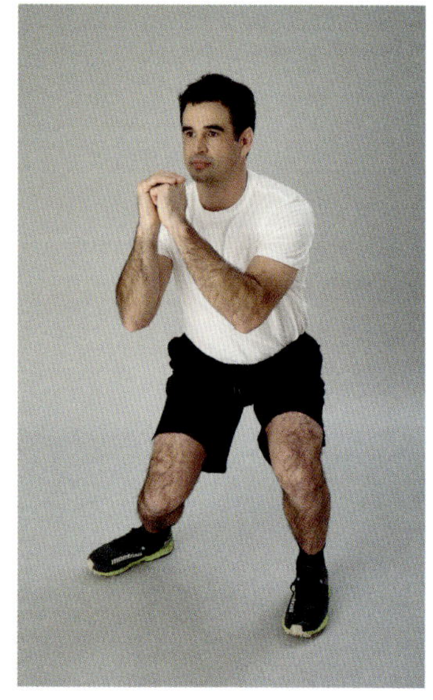

Starting position

Stand with your feet a little wider than shoulder-width apart, toes facing outward slightly, arms clasped in front of your chest. Squat down and hold.

The movement

Shift your weight from one leg to the other to momentarily perform a bit of a single-leg squat. Shift back and forth several times before standing up.

Tip: Keep your weight-bearing knee, foot, and shin directly under you when you shift over to each leg.

Deep Goblet Squats

EQUIPMENT: Moderate to heavy dumbbell

2 SETS OF 6–8 REPS

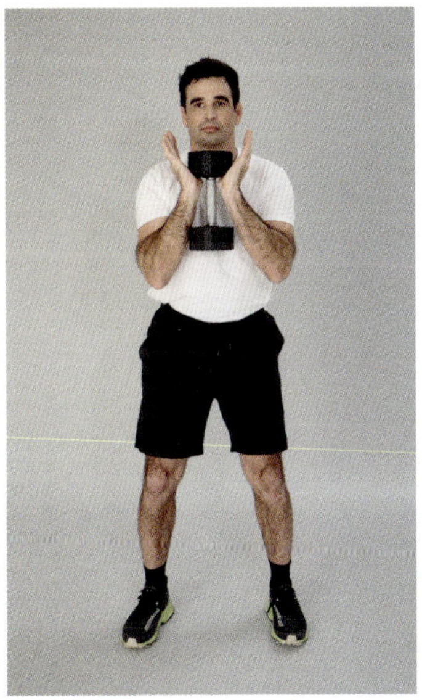 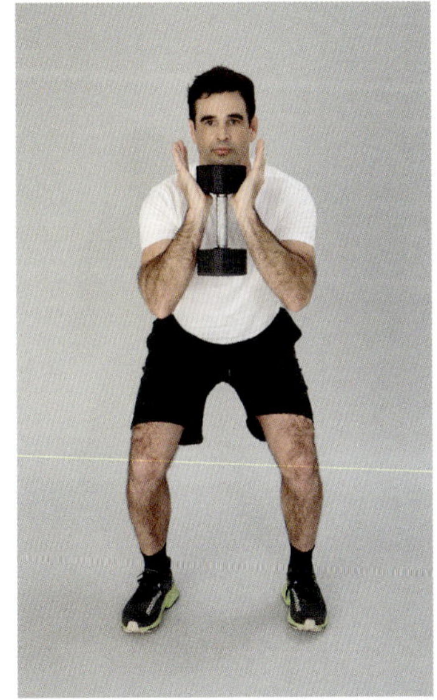 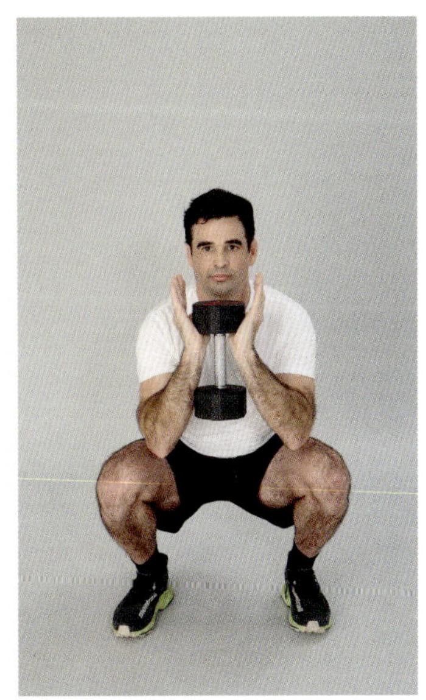

Starting position

Stand with feet slightly wider than shoulder-width apart, toes pointed outward. Hold the dumbbell vertically with your hands wrapped around the top head to form a goblet shape.

The movement

Push your hips back, and let your knees track over your toes as you lower your hips between your feet and your elbows between your knees. Press into your heels to stand up.

Tip: Keep your forearms as vertical as possible so you don't bend forward too much and fatigue your arms.

ROUTINE #3

WIDE SQUATS

3 sets of 12–20 reps

HIP SWEEPS

2 sets of 3 reps each side

WALKING LUNGES

14–30 reps or for distance

SUSPENSION HAMSTRING CURLS

2 sets of 8–12 reps

LATERAL SKIP SQUATS

2 sets of 12–20 reps

Wide Squats

EQUIPMENT: Dumbbell (optional)

3 SETS OF 12–20 REPS

Starting position

Stand with feet about two shoulder widths apart, toes pointing outward slightly. If using a dumbbell, hold it vertically with your hands wrapped around the top head to form a goblet shape.

The movement

Push your hips back, and bend your knees over your toes to squat down as low as your mobility will allow. Pause, then stand up.

Tip: For balance, lift your arms in front of you as you descend.

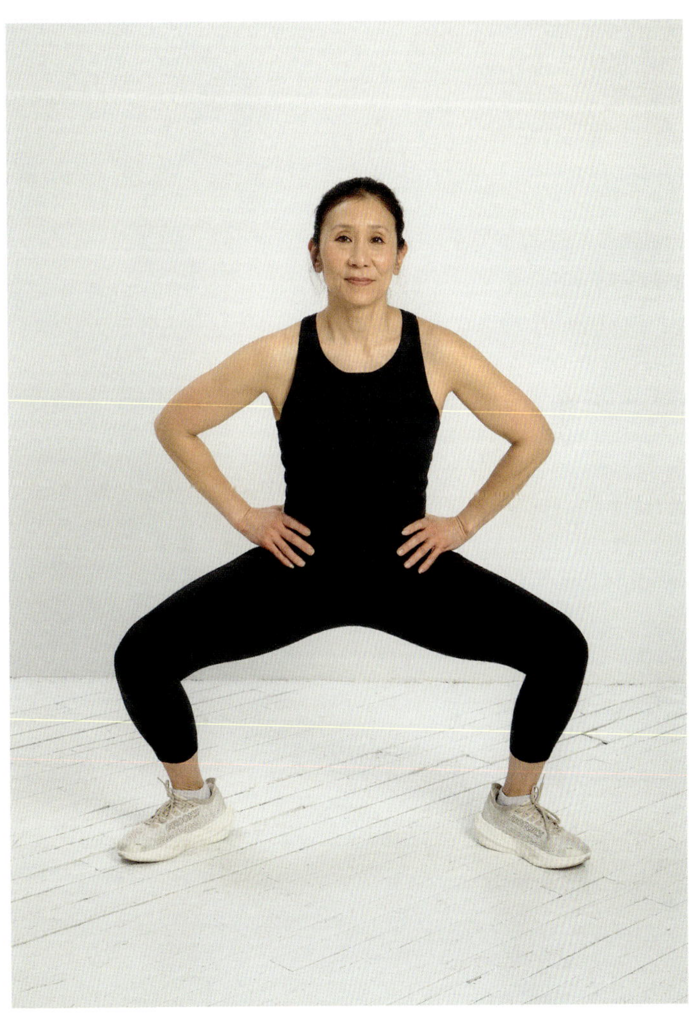

Hip Sweeps

EQUIPMENT: Wall or sturdy table for support

2 SETS OF 3 REPS EACH SIDE

Starting position

Stand, and lift one leg straight out in front of you, keeping both legs straight.

The movement

Swing the lifted leg out to your side, and continue the rotation until it's behind you. Pause, then sweep the leg to the front, and lower it to the ground. Try to keep both legs straight the whole time.

Tip: Lift the leg higher to make this more difficult or keep it low to focus on stability.

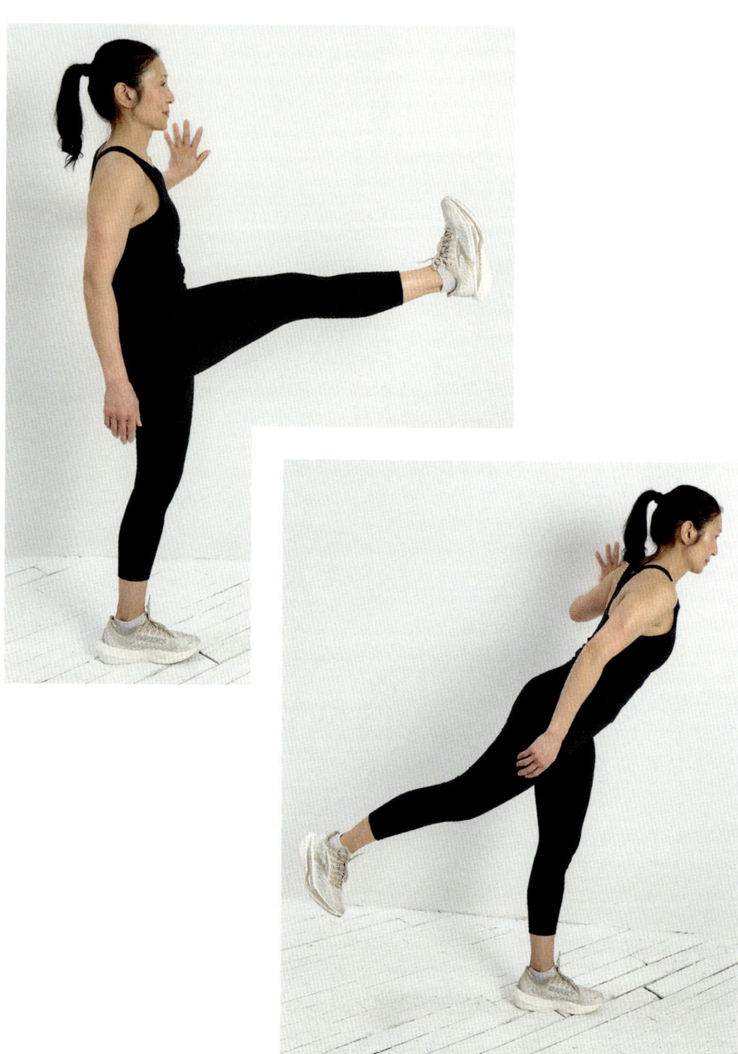

Walking Lunges

EQUIPMENT: 2 dumbbells (optional)

14–30 REPS OR FOR DISTANCE

Starting position

In an indoor or outdoor space with lots of room to walk, stand with both feet together and hands on your hips or clasped in front of your chest. If using dumbbells, hold them down by your sides.

The movement

Take a big step forward, placing most of your weight on your front heel. Squat down, pulling your hip closer to your front heel with your knee tracking over your toes. Pause, hovering an inch off the ground or touching the ground with one knee, then pull yourself back to a standing position with the front leg. Repeat, alternating legs.

Tip: Tilt your torso forward to match the angle of your shin to improve stability and hip strength.

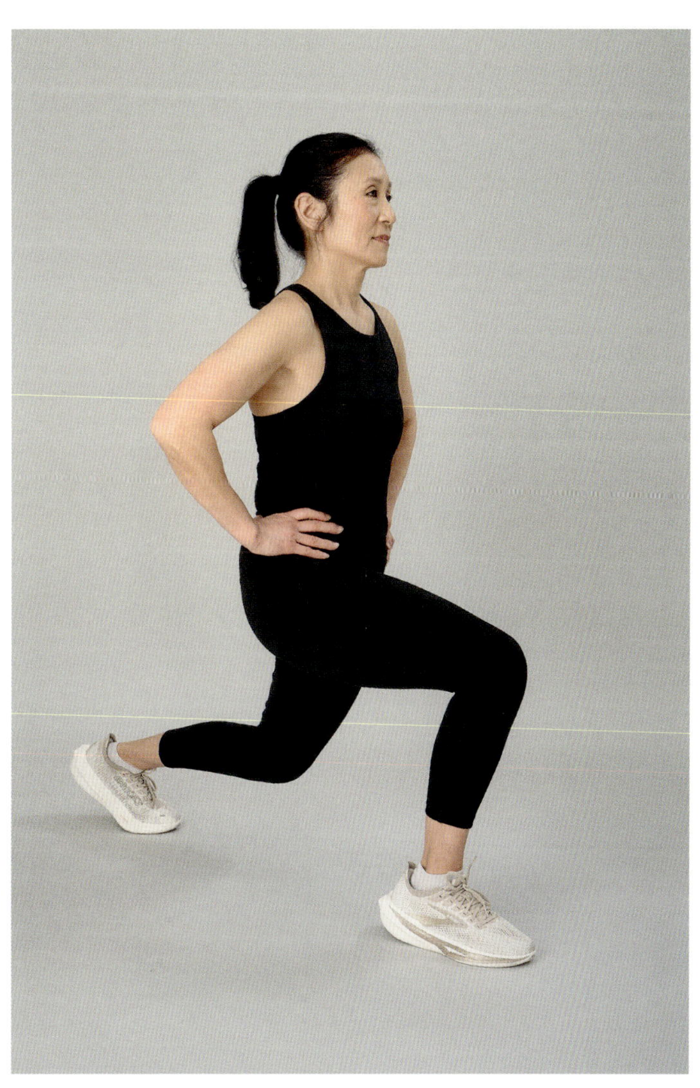

Suspension Hamstring Curls

EQUIPMENT: Suspension straps attached to overhead support or door anchor, exercise mat or rug for support (optional)

2 SETS OF 8–12 REPS

Starting position

Lie on your back on the floor with your heels in the straps' foot loops at about knee height. Clench your glutes to lift your hips off the floor.

The movement

Pull your heels back toward your hips while lifting your hips to keep your body as straight as possible.

Tip: Keep your back squeezed in toward your spine with palms facing up to provide support along your entire posterior chain.

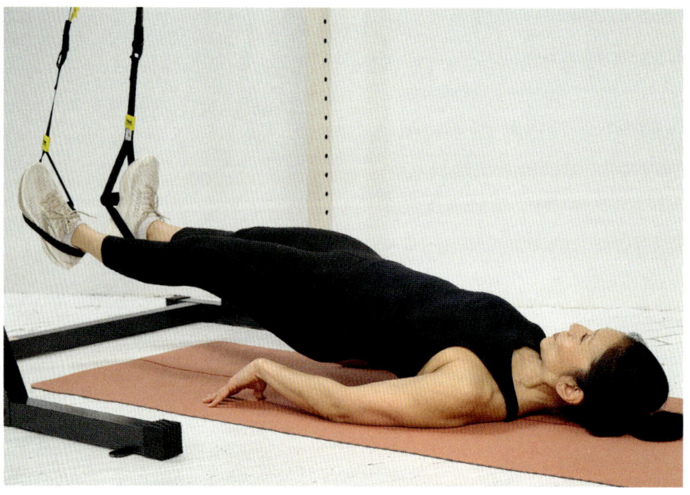

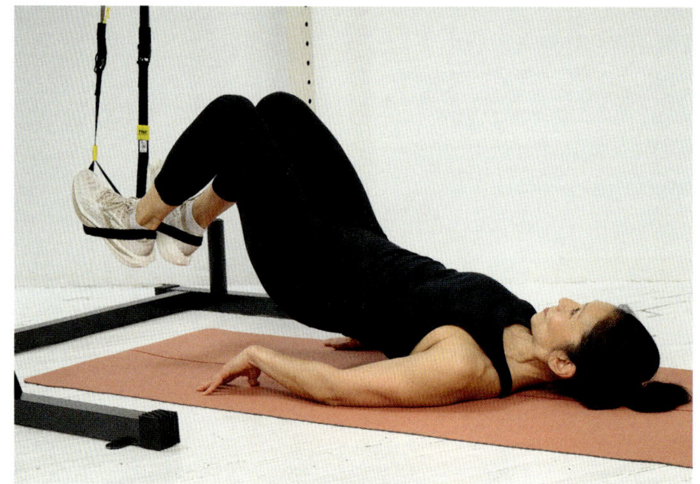

Lateral Skip Squats

EQUIPMENT: None

2 SETS OF 12–20 REPS

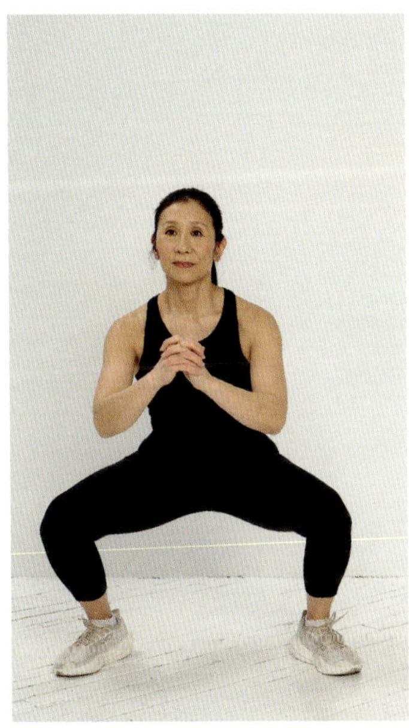

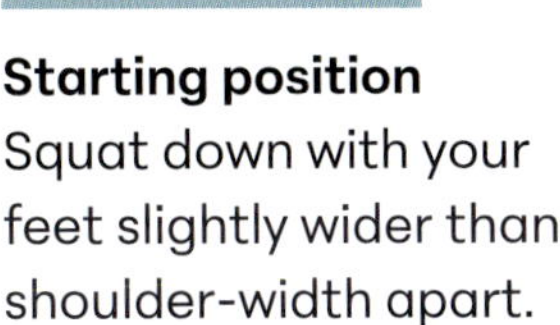

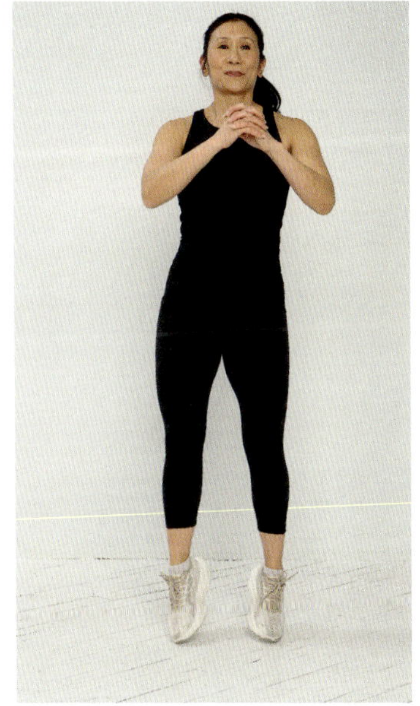

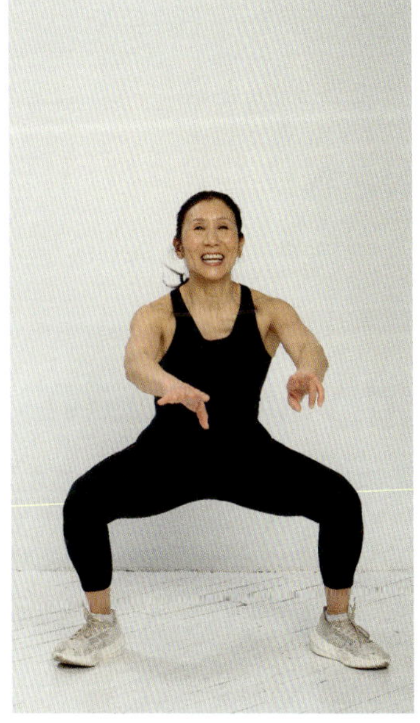

Starting position

Squat down with your feet slightly wider than shoulder-width apart.

The movement

Stand, and skip to the side by clicking your feet together lightly before landing into a moderately wide squat. Repeat in a continuous motion for distance or back and forth.

Tip: Make this more difficult by jumping higher during the skip and squatting deeper on the landing.

ROUTINE #4

BAND DEADLIFT

3 sets of 12–15 reps

REVERSE LUNGES

2 sets of 20–30 reps each leg

STANDING CALF RAISES

2 sets of 20 reps

NARROW SQUATS

2 sets of 12 reps

SKATER SQUATS

2 sets of 20 reps

Band Deadlift

EQUIPMENT: Heavy resistance band

3 SETS OF 12–15 REPS

Starting position

Stand with feet about shoulder width and a half apart, with one end of the band around each midfoot. Hinge forward, and grab both the top and bottom of the band.

The movement

Drive your hips forward, and use your glutes and hamstrings to stand upright while pulling your shoulders back to keep your back straight. Reverse the movement to lower again to starting position.

Tip: Try not to lean back at the top. Think of standing up in a tall posture.

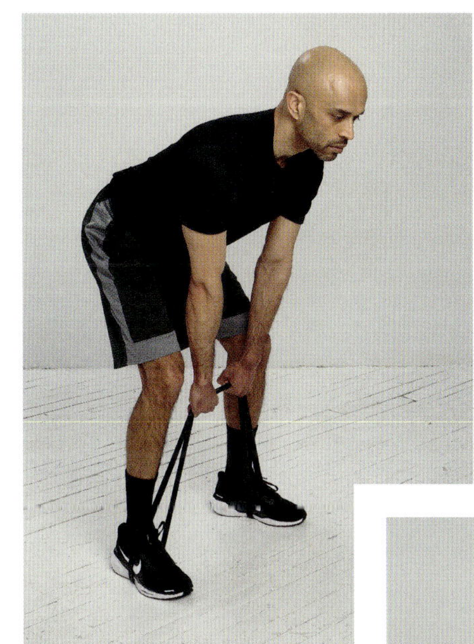

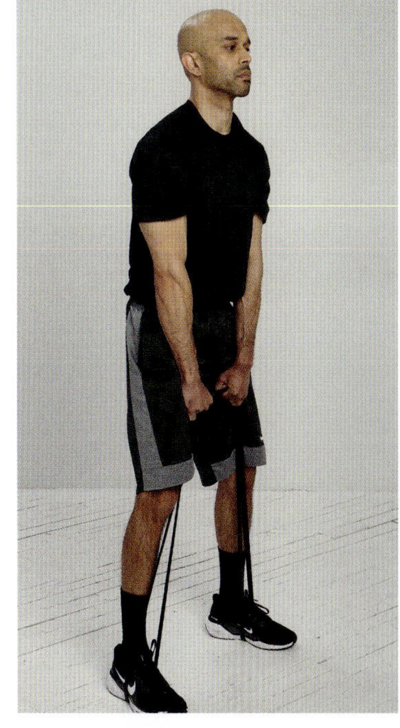

Reverse Lunges

EQUIPMENT: 2 moderate to heavy dumbbells (optional)

2 SETS OF 20–30 REPS EACH LEG

Starting position

Stand with feet together and hands on hips. If using dumbbells, hold them down by your sides.

The movement

Step one foot back while keeping your weight on your front leg. Squat down on the front leg, tracking your knee over your toes and bringing your back knee about 1 inch above the floor. Stand back up, pulling your back leg back to starting position.

Tip: Keep your weight on the front foot throughout the exercise, and avoid shifting too much weight to the back foot as you step back.

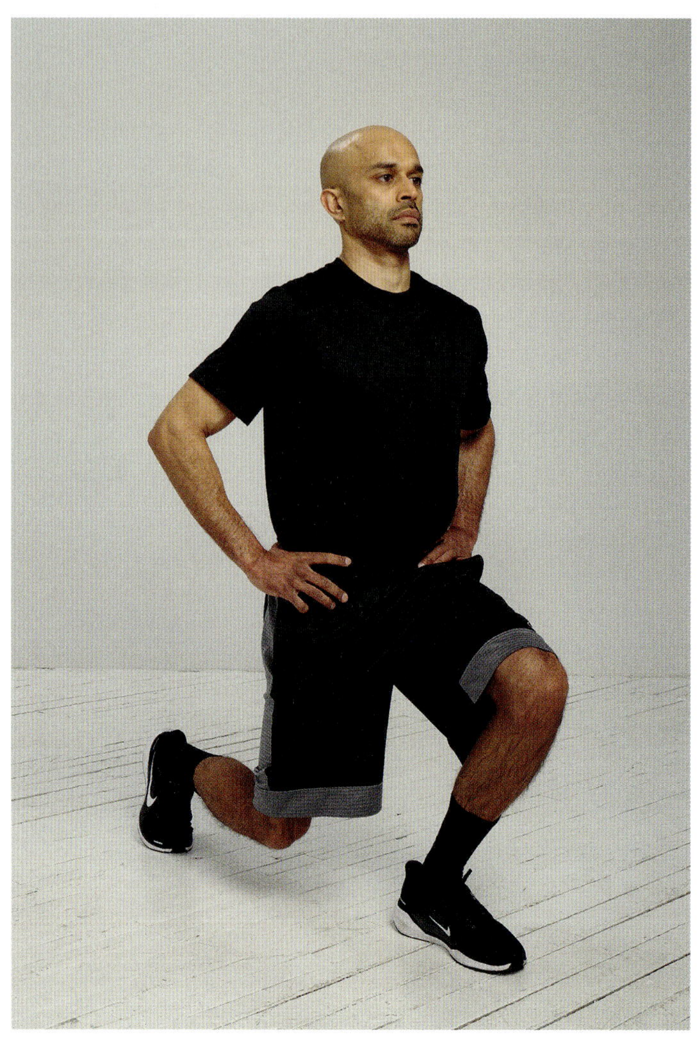

ROUTINE #4   LOWER BODY

Standing Calf Raises

EQUIPMENT: Wall or countertop for support (optional)

2 SETS OF 20 REPS

Starting position

Stand with feet about 6 inches apart. Place one hand on a wall or countertop for support, if needed.

The movement

Press down into the balls of your feet to lift your heels as high as possible. Pause, then lower down under control without letting your weight shift to your heels.

Tip: Keep all of your leg muscles tense, including your hamstrings, glutes, and quads (fronts of thighs), to maintain strict technique.

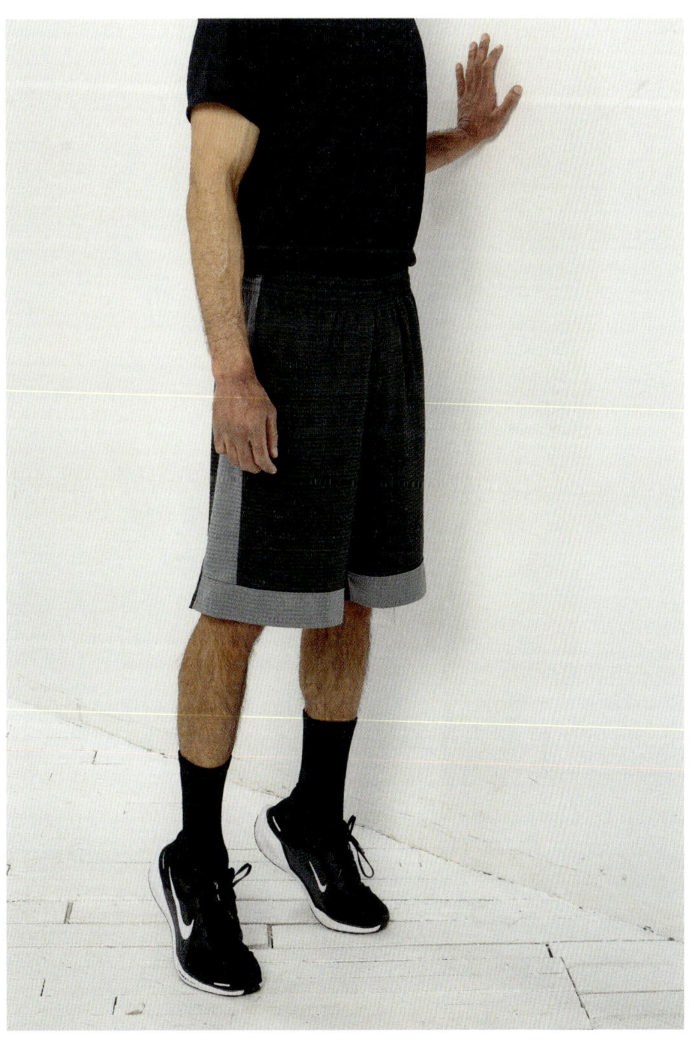

Narrow Squats

EQUIPMENT: Light dumbbell (optional)

2 SETS OF 12 REPS

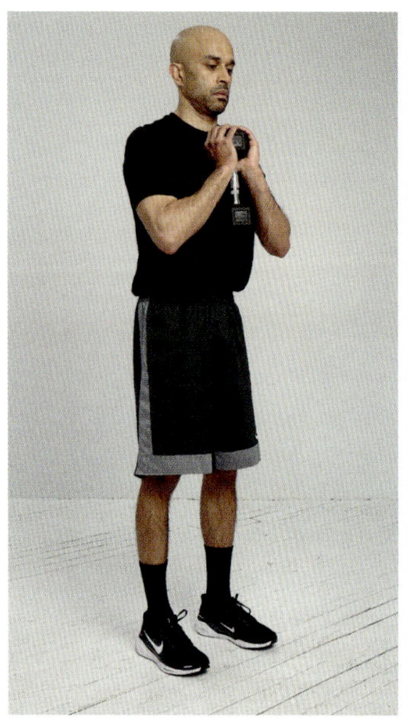 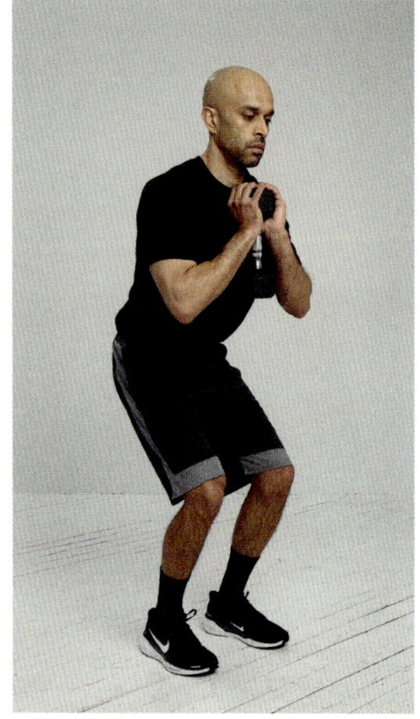 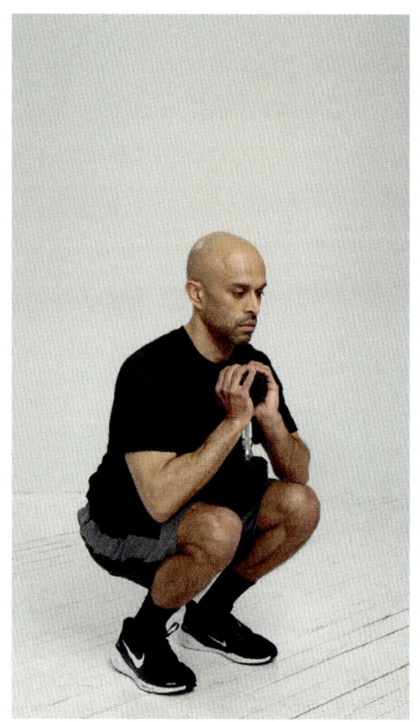

Starting position

Stand with your feet about 6 inches apart and hands down by your sides. If using a dumbbell, hold it vertically positioned at your collarbone, with your hands wrapped around the top head to form a goblet shape.

The movement

Squat down by pushing your hips back and letting your knees track forward over your toes. If not using a dumbbell, lift your arms in front of you to maintain stability and allow for more depth in the squat.

Tip: Think about stretching your hips as you squat down to improve mobility and control.

Skater Squats

EQUIPMENT: None

2 SETS OF 20 REPS

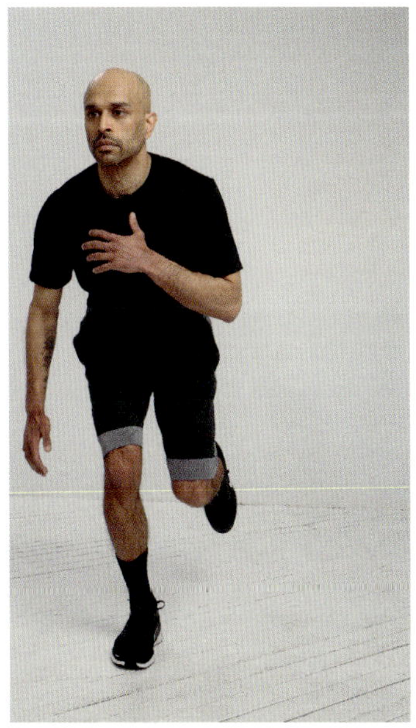 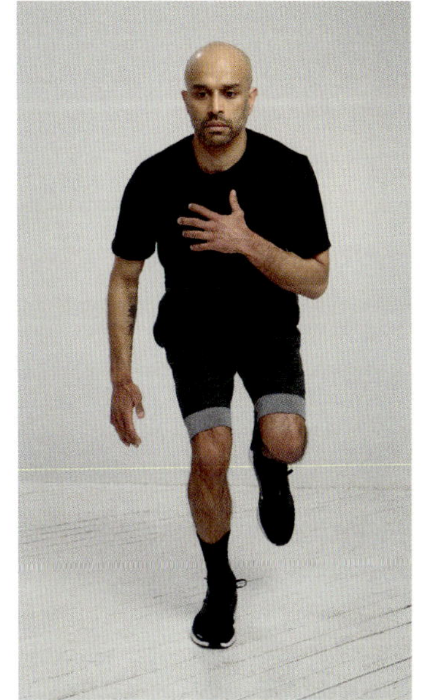 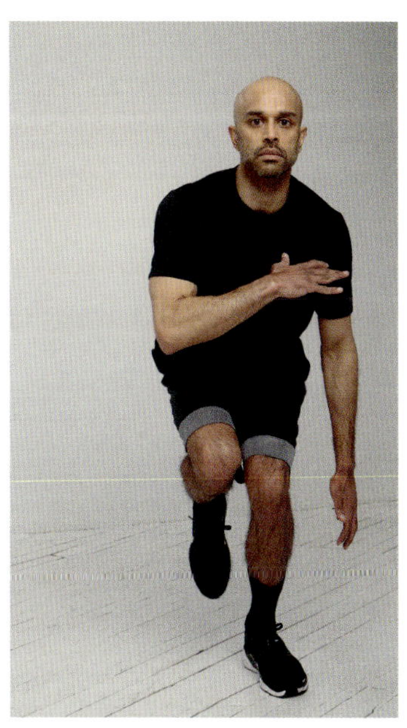

Starting position
Stand on one leg, lifting the other leg slightly, and bend the supporting leg into a short squat.

The movement
Jump a few feet to the side of the bent leg (toward the lifted leg), and land into a one-leg squat with the opposite (lifted) leg. Repeat, alternating legs.

Tip: Adjust the difficulty with how high and far you jump as well as how deep you squat.

CHAPTER 5

Core

Have you ever tried to crush a chicken egg in your hand? Despite its perceived fragility, you cannot crack an egg in one hand no matter how hard you squeeze it. The human body works in much the same way. You can withstand an incredible amount of force and stress—when it's applied in a balanced way. Conversely, the body can break down easily when even the slightest pressure is applied under the wrong circumstances.

Martial arts practitioners understand this concept. A skilled martial artist can break through concrete using their bare hands. The key to how this works is alignment. Your body can withstand loads of force as long as that force is allowed to travel through your body like electricity. The problem arises when that force can't travel through your body and, instead, creates localized pressure in the joints.

The exercises in this chapter are designed to promote strength and the smooth transfer of force through your body. They condition your fundamental and anatomical chains collectively known as "the core." Many of these exercises engage your muscles isometrically; that is, through resistance without stretching or contracting, so there's no movement happening with your body. Isometric strength training is very effective for building strength and avoiding stress in the hips and lower back.

Core training is often considered effective for strengthening the abdominals and obliques, but it also works your hips, hamstrings, and the delicate muscles that run along your spine. Conditioning these muscles with the exercises and techniques in this chapter will promote the proper alignment to build lifelong resilience, as well as improve the effectiveness of your upper and lower body training from the previous chapters. The exercises that follow take a holistic approach that, in addition to improving your full-body strength, will help you look and feel your best by improving your posture—truly at the core of it all.

ROUTINE #1

CAT-COW

12–15 reps

LATERAL SIDE PRESS

2 sets for 10–15 seconds each side

TABLE PRESS

2 sets for 10–15 seconds each

WALL KICK-BACK

3 sets for 15 seconds each leg

STANDING TWIST

2 sets for 10 seconds each side

Cat-Cow

EQUIPMENT: Exercise mat or rug for support

12–15 REPS

Starting position
Place your hands on the floor under your shoulders and your knees under your hips in a crawling position.

The movement
Arch your back up into a "cat" position by looking down, crunching your abs, and pushing your shoulders forward so your back is rounded at the top. Then, reverse the motion, arching your back down into a "cow" position, turning your gaze upward.

Tip: Actively squeeze the floor between your hands and knees to maintain tension in your abdominals throughout the movement.

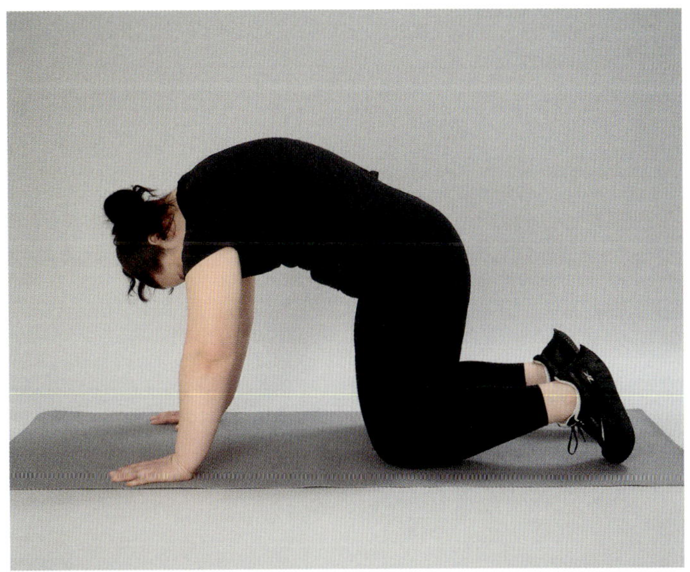

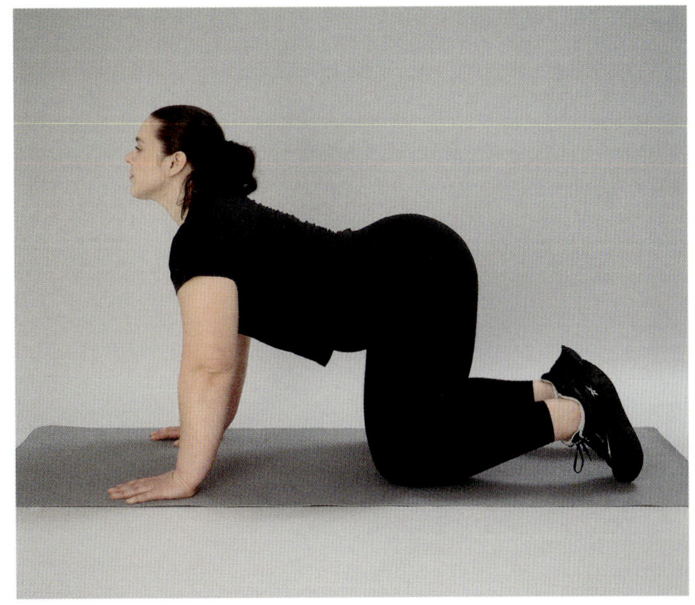

Lateral Side Press

EQUIPMENT: Countertop or suspension straps at about waist height

2 SETS FOR 10–15 SECONDS EACH SIDE

Starting position

Standing sideways to the counter, hold your arm straight out to the side, and place your palm on the counter. Keep your weight on the leg closest to the counter.

The movement

Use the muscles along the side of your body to isometrically press your palm downward. Hold, then repeat on the other side.

Tip: Keep your abdominals and hips tight to prevent shifting your pelvis away from the countertop while pressing.

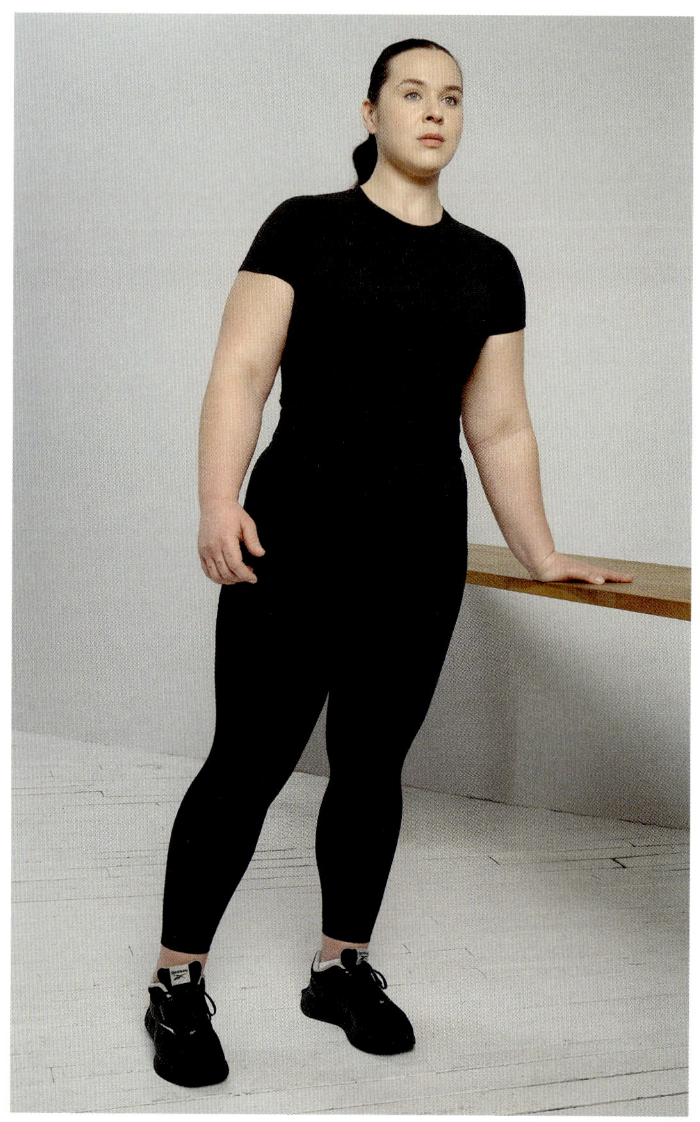

Table Press

EQUIPMENT: Countertop or suspension straps at about waist height

2 SETS FOR 10–15 SECONDS EACH

Starting position

Face the countertop with your arms stretched out in front of you and hands resting on the counter. Arch your back slightly, rounding it like in the "cat" position (see page 105).

The movement

Contract all of the muscles along the front of your body to isometrically press your hands down into the countertop.

Tip: Keep your breathing smooth and steady throughout the exercise.

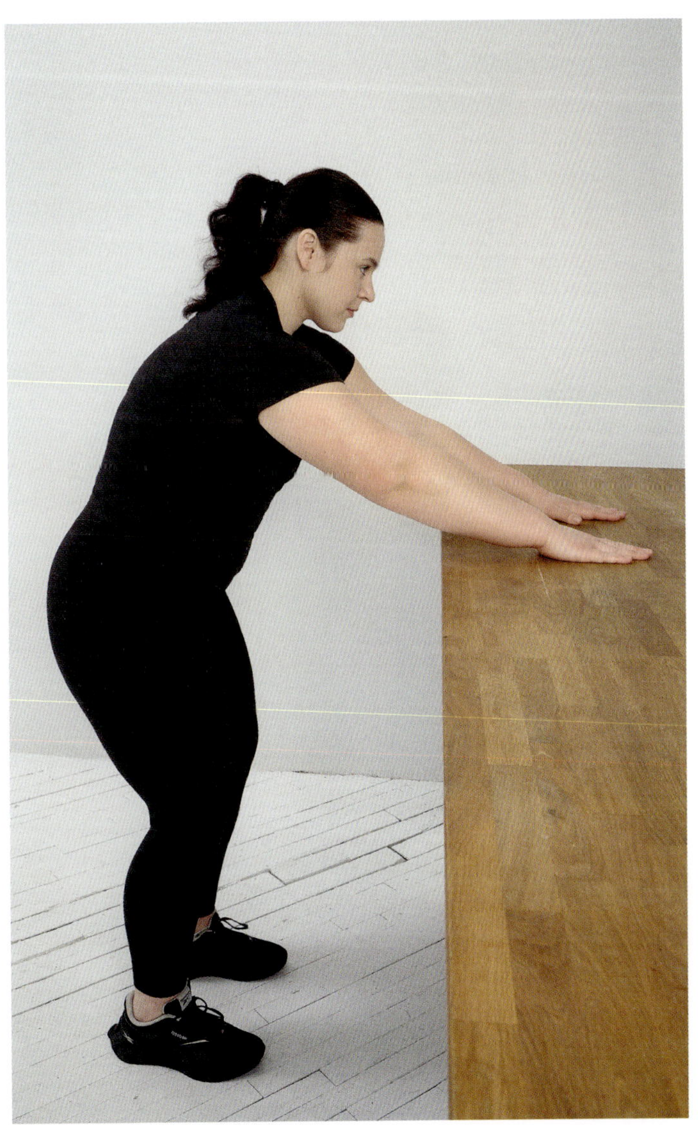

Wall Kick-Back

EQUIPMENT: Wall

3 SETS FOR 15 SECONDS EACH LEG

Starting position
Stand about 18 inches away from the wall with your back to the wall. Place the back of your heel against the wall while keeping your legs straight.

The movement
Use the muscles along the back of your leg to isometrically press your heel against the wall. Alternate feet, and repeat on the other side.

Tip: Lean your torso forward slightly so it's roughly the same angle as your rear leg to make sure your hips do the work and not your lower back.

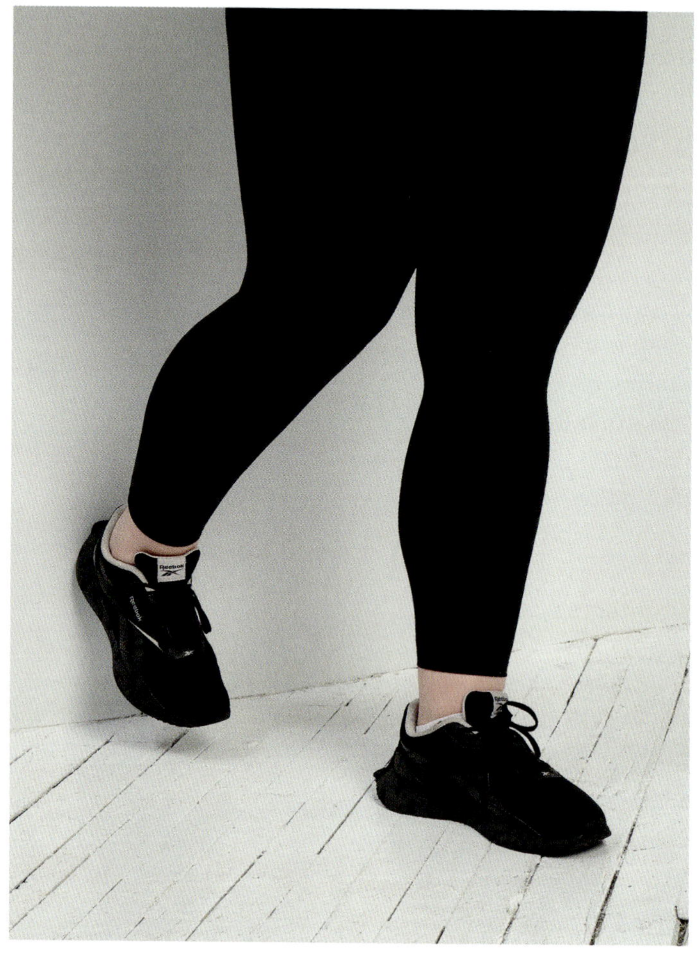

Standing Twist

EQUIPMENT: None

2 SETS FOR 10 SECONDS EACH SIDE

Starting position
Standing upright, place the back of one hand against your lower back and the opposite hand across your chest and on your shoulder.

The movement
Turn your head to look, and twist your torso toward the hand on your shoulder. Hold, then repeat on the other side.

Tip: Avoid rotating at your hips to emphasize the strength and mobility along your spine.

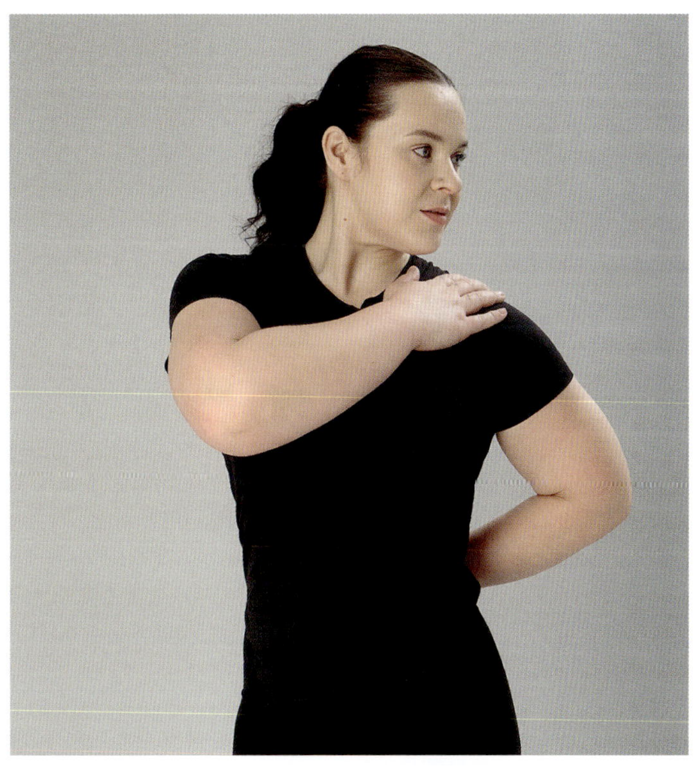

ROUTINE #2

DEAD BUG

3 sets for 10–15 seconds

BEAR PLANK

3 sets for 15 seconds

SEATED TWIST STRETCH

2 sets for 20 seconds each side

LYING HIP BRIDGE

3 sets of 15–20 reps

LYING KNEE RAISE

2 sets of 10–15 reps

Dead Bug

EQUIPMENT: Exercise mat or rug for support

3 SETS FOR 10–15 SECONDS

Starting position

Lying on your back, bend and lift your legs so your calves are parallel to the floor. Place your forearms against your thighs, with your back rounded slightly. Tuck your chin to your chest.

The movement

Isometrically contract your abs to push your arms and legs together as hard as you can.

Tip: As you engage, be sure to breathe with long, continuous breaths.

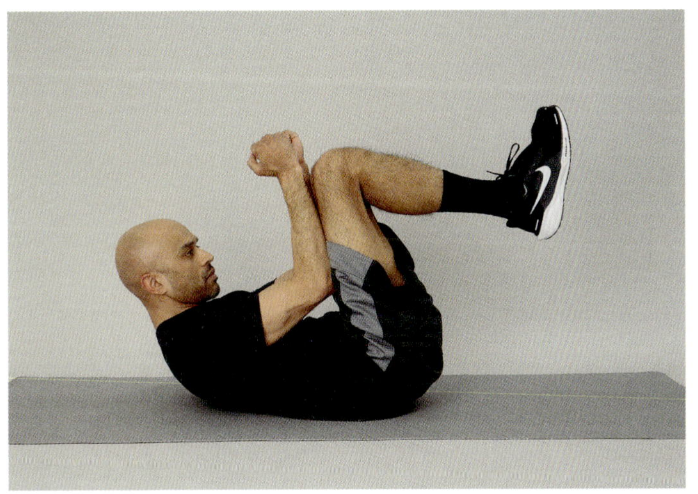

Bear Plank

EQUIPMENT: Exercise mat or rug for support

3 SETS FOR 15 SECONDS

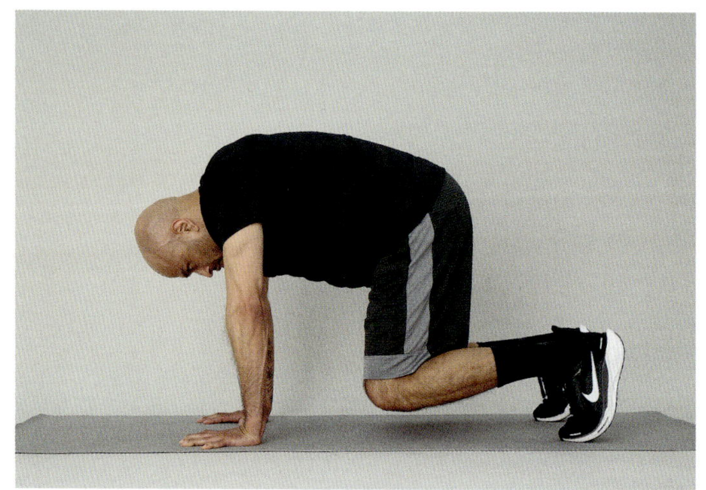

Starting position

Place your hands on the floor under your shoulders and your knees under your hips in a crawling position.

The movement

Arch your back up into a "cat" position by looking down, crunching your abs, and pushing your shoulders forward so your back is rounded at the top. Lift your knees 2 inches off the floor while continuing to squeeze the floor between your hands and your toes.

Tip: Flex your abdominals before lifting your legs to avoid pressure in your lower back.

Seated Twist Stretch

EQUIPMENT: Exercise mat or rug for support

2 SETS FOR 20 SECONDS EACH SIDE

Starting position

Sit on the floor with your legs straight out in front of you. Bend your right leg over your straight left leg and put your right foot against the outside of your left knee. Place your left arm on the outside of your bent knee and your right hand on the ground behind you for support.

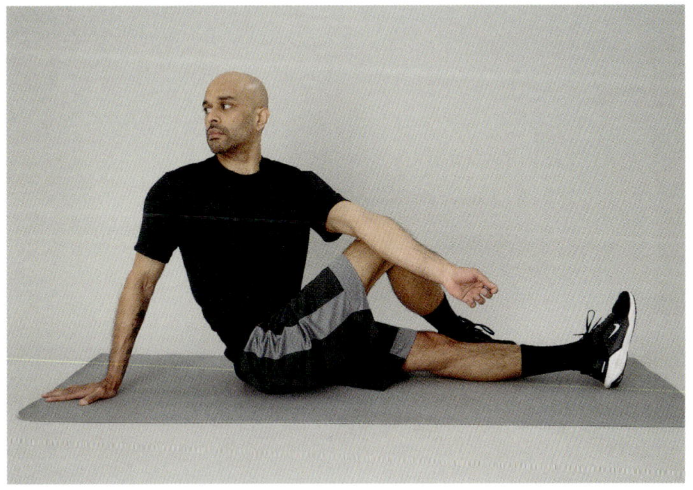

The movement

Turn your head to the right. Apply pressure against your bent knee with your left arm; hold. Repeat on the other side.

Tip: Sit up as straight as possible to improve posture and minimize stress along your spine.

Lying Hip Bridge

EQUIPMENT: Exercise mat or rug for support

3 SETS OF 15–20 REPS

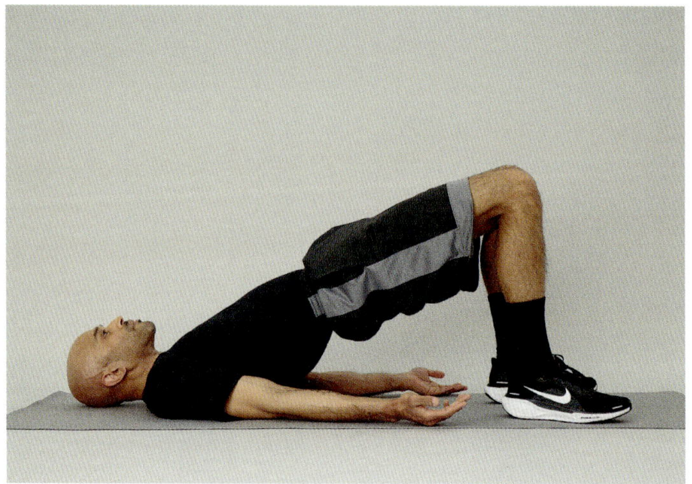

Starting position

Lie on your back with your knees bent and feet flat on the floor. Place your hands by your sides, palms facing up.

The movement

Press into your heels, and tense your glutes to lift your hips upward. Pause at the top, then lower under control.

Tip: Pull into your heels, and maintain tension in your glutes throughout the full range of motion to avoid using your lower back.

Lying Knee Raise

EQUIPMENT: Exercise mat or rug for support

2 SETS OF 10–15 REPS

Starting position

Lie on your back with your knees bent and feet flat on the floor. Place your hands by your side, palms facing down.

The movement

Contract your abdominals to lift your knees toward your chest, allowing your hips to roll up off the floor. Pause at the top, then lower your feet under control.

Tip: Maintain tension in your quads so your abdominals stay tense throughout the full range of motion.

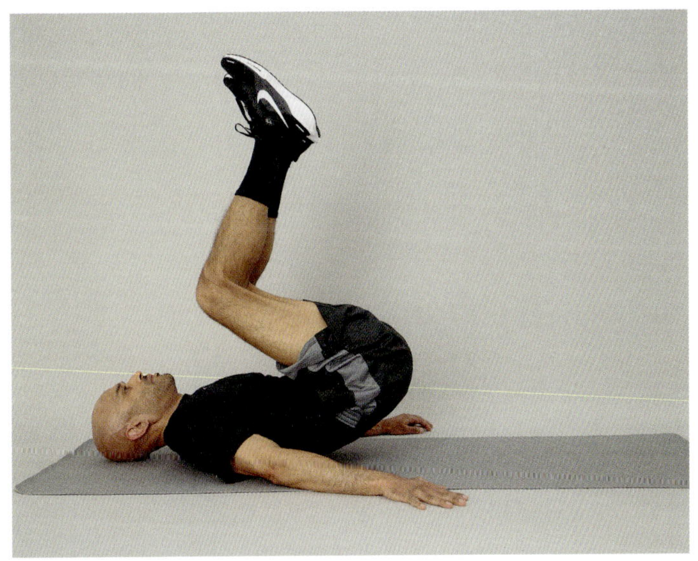

ROUTINE #3

HOLLOW-BODY PLANK

2 holds for 20–30 seconds each

RUSSIAN TWIST

2 sets of 20 reps

SIDE PLANK ON KNEES

2 holds for 10–15 seconds each side

ELEVATED LYING HIP BRIDGE

3 sets of 15–20 reps

LYING LEG RAISES

2 sets of 10–12 reps

Hollow-Body Plank

EQUIPMENT: Exercise mat or rug for support

2 HOLDS FOR 20–30 SECONDS EACH

Starting position

Place your hands on the floor under your shoulders and your knees under your hips in a crawling position. Arch your back up into a "cat" position by looking down, crunching your abs, and pushing your shoulders forward so your back is rounded at the top.

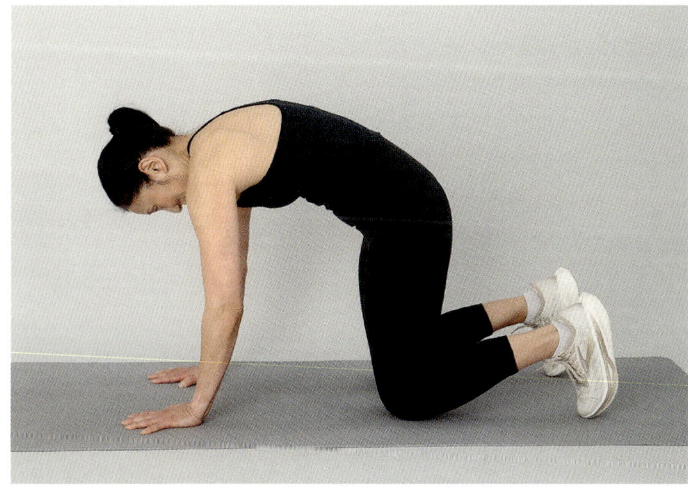

The movement

Extend both legs behind you, lifting your knees while maintaining the arch in your back; hold.

Tip: Maintain tension in your glutes and quads to support your hips and avoid stress in your lower back.

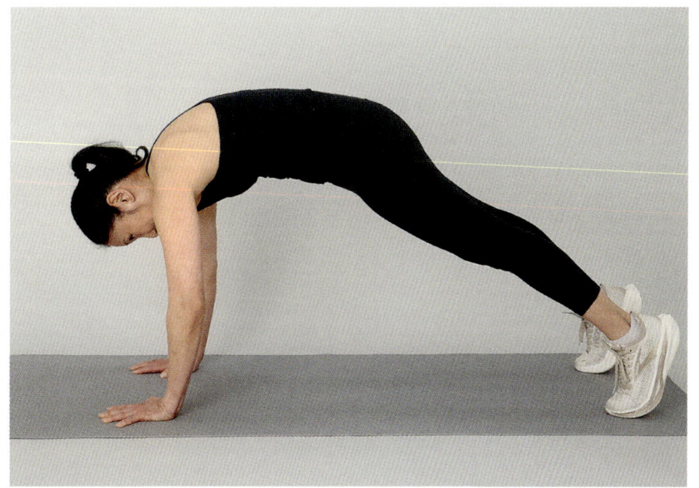

Russian Twist

EQUIPMENT: Exercise mat or rug for support, light dumbbell (optional)

2 SETS OF 20 REPS

Starting position

Sit on the floor with your knees bent, and lean back slightly. Place your hands together at your chest, or hold a dumbbell just below your chest.

The movement

Twist to one side while reaching both hands toward the floor. Hold for 2 seconds, then twist to the other side.

Tip: Lean back farther to add resistance, or sit up more to make the exercise easier.

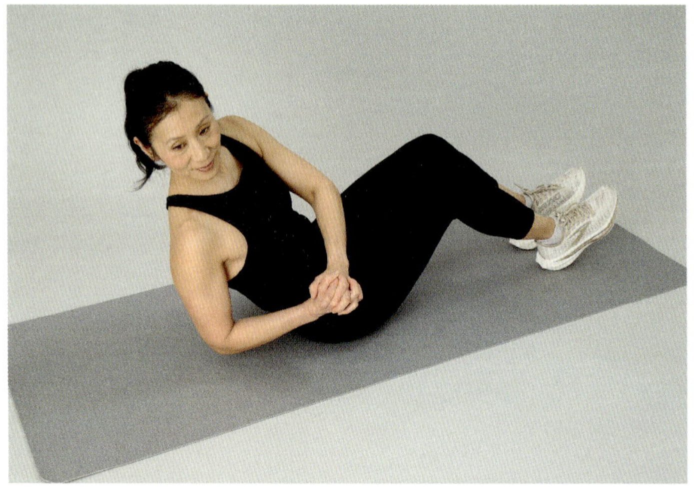

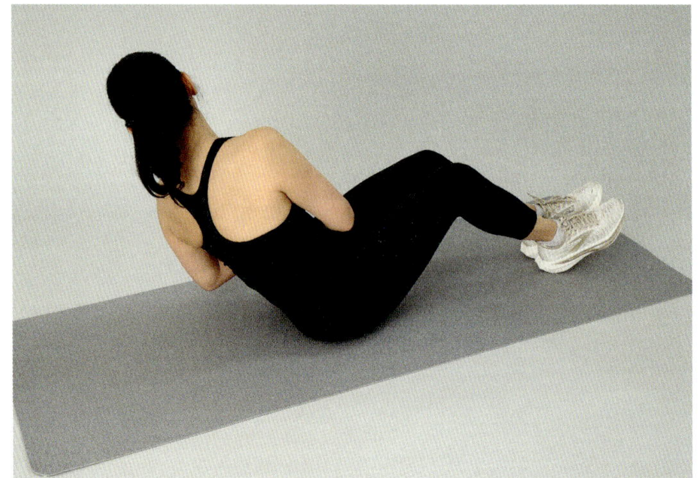

Side Plank on Knees

EQUIPMENT: Exercise mat or rug for support

2 HOLDS FOR 10–15 SECONDS EACH SIDE

Starting position

Lie on your side, supporting yourself on your forearm, with knees bent at a 90-degree angle and feet behind you.

The movement

Lift your hips to form a straight line between the top of your head and your knees on the floor. Hold, then repeat on the other side.

Tip: Clench your glutes to push your hips forward. This will ensure more total tension throughout the front and back side of your lateral (side) core muscles.

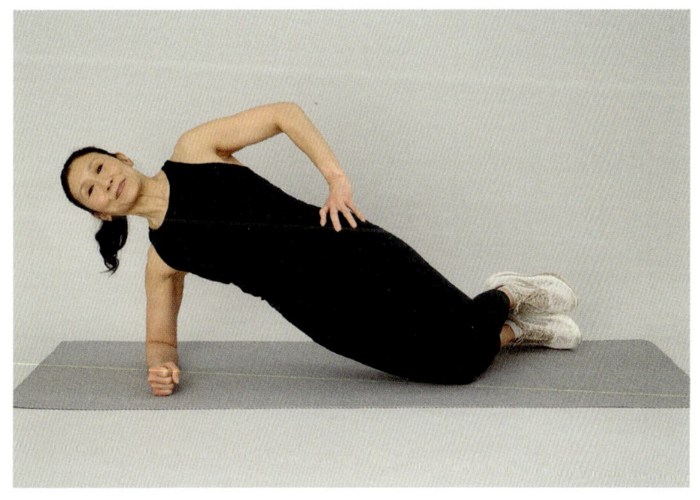

Elevated Lying Hip Bridge

EQUIPMENT: Exercise mat or rug for support, sturdy chair

3 SETS OF 15–20 REPS

Starting position

Lie on your back with the backs of your heels resting on the chair seat and knees bent at a 90-degree angle. Place your palms face down by your sides.

The movement

Tense your glutes and hamstrings to press the backs of your heels into the chair and lift your hips upward. Pause at the top, then lower your hips under control.

Tip: Press into your heels to maintain tension in your hamstrings.

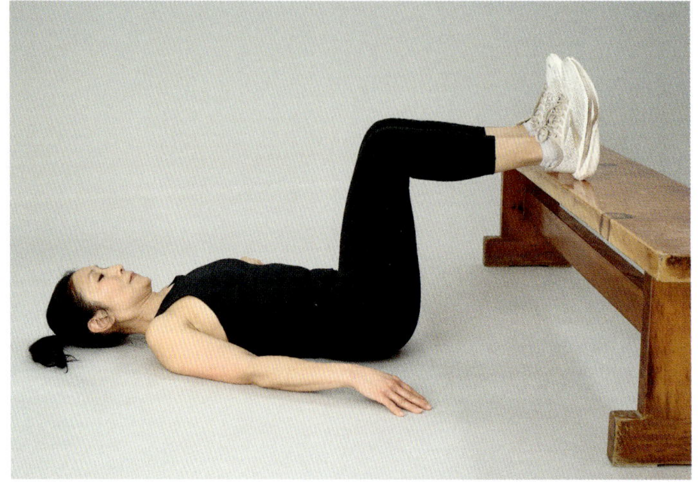

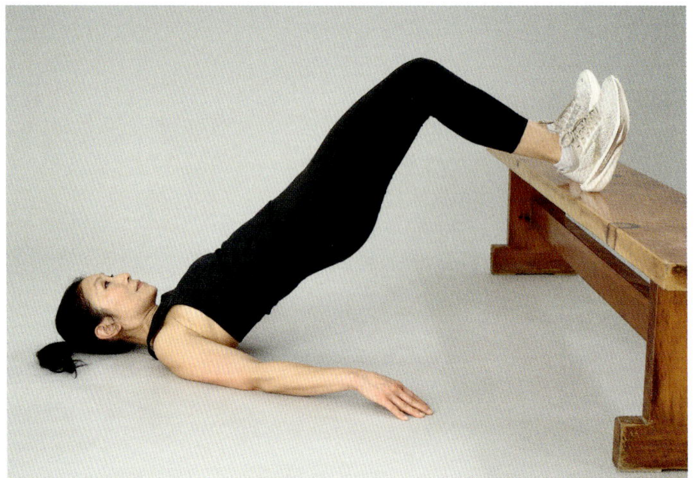

Lying Leg Raises

EQUIPMENT: Exercise mat or rug for support

2 SETS OF 10–12 REPS

Starting position

Lie on your back with your legs flat on the floor and palms facing down by your sides.

The movement

Tense your abdominals to press your lower back onto the floor, then lift your legs straight up in a controlled motion. Lower the legs, and lightly touch your heels on the floor.

Tip: Bend your knees slightly to reduce resistance, or lock your legs straight to build more strength and mobility.

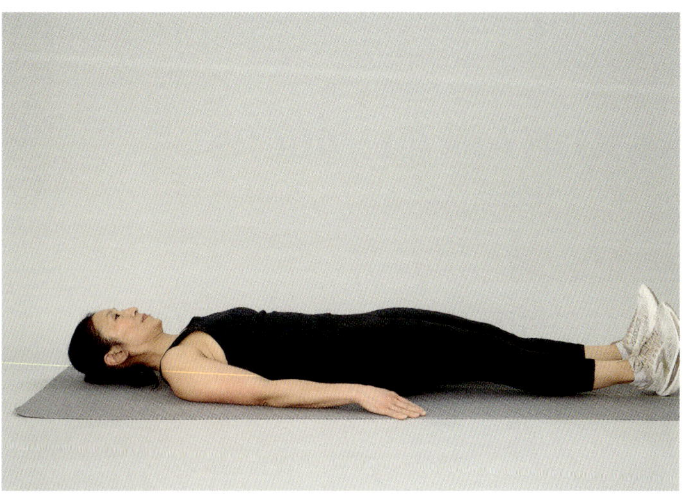

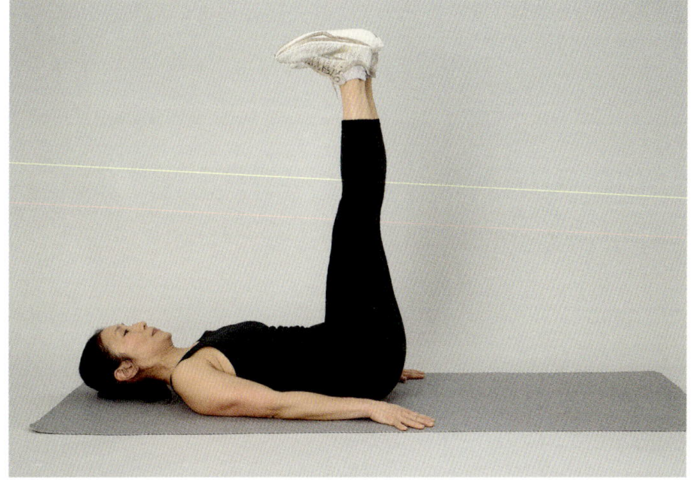

ROUTINE #4

MOUNTAIN CLIMBERS

2 sets of 8–10 each leg

SEATED LATERAL LEG LIFTS

2 sets of 12–14 reps

TABLE BRIDGE

2 sets of 12–15 reps

SIDE PLANK WITH HIP LIFTS

2 sets of 12–20 reps each side

V-SITS

2 sets of 12–16 reps

Mountain Climbers

EQUIPMENT: Exercise mat or rug for support

2 SETS OF 8–10 EACH LEG

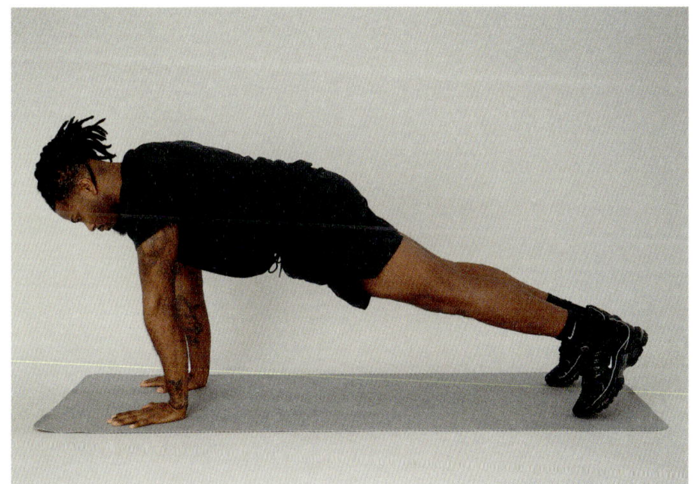

Starting position

Set up in a plank position (see page 26), placing hands and toes on the floor and rounding your back slightly.

The movement

Tuck one knee up toward your chest while lifting your hips slightly in a smooth and controlled motion. Pause, and let your hips drop slightly when you return the foot to the ground. Repeat on the other side.

Tip: Keep pressing your shoulders forward throughout the exercise to provide upper-body stability.

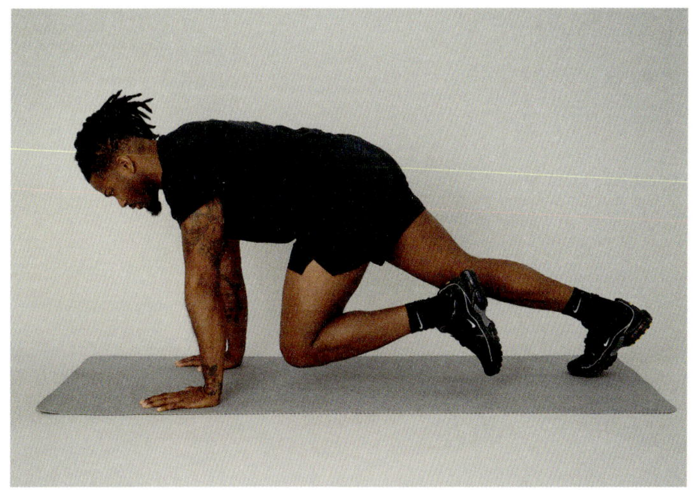

Seated Lateral Leg Lifts

EQUIPMENT: Exercise mat or rug for support, dumbell or object about 8 inches high (optional)

2 SETS OF 12–14 REPS

Starting position

In a seated position on the floor, lean back with your legs straight out in front of you and angled slightly to one side. Place your hands on the ground behind you for support, or hold them in front of your chest for added difficulty.

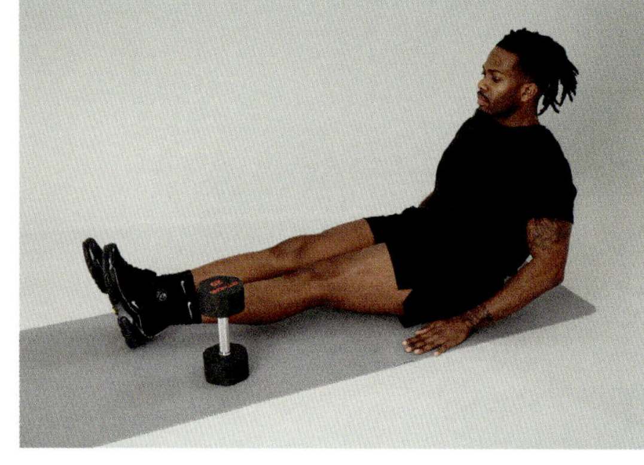

The movement

Lift your legs up and over to the other side in an arching rainbow movement.

Tip: Place an object (such as a dumbbell on its side) by your feet to challenge yourself to lift the legs over it.

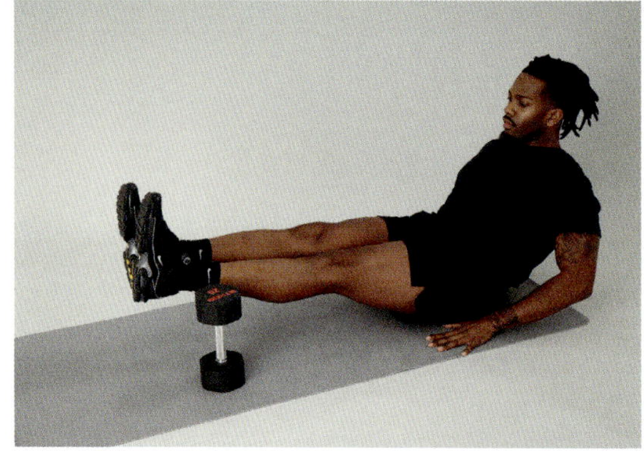

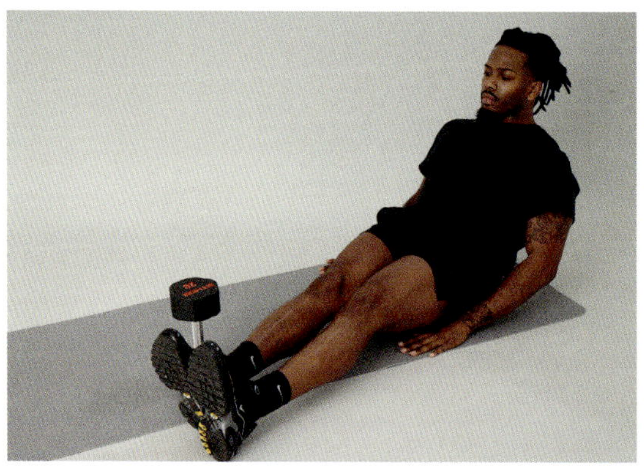

Table Bridge

EQUIPMENT: Exercise mat or rug for support (something with traction for your hands and feet)
2 SETS OF 12–15 REPS

Starting position
Sit with your hands behind you and knees bent at a 90-degree angle, heels on the ground.

The movement
Tense your glutes and hamstrings to lift your hips into a "table" position with feet on the ground. Pause, then lower down while maintaining tension in the hips.

Tip: Roll your shoulders back, and lift your chest high before each rep to ensure proper support along your spine.

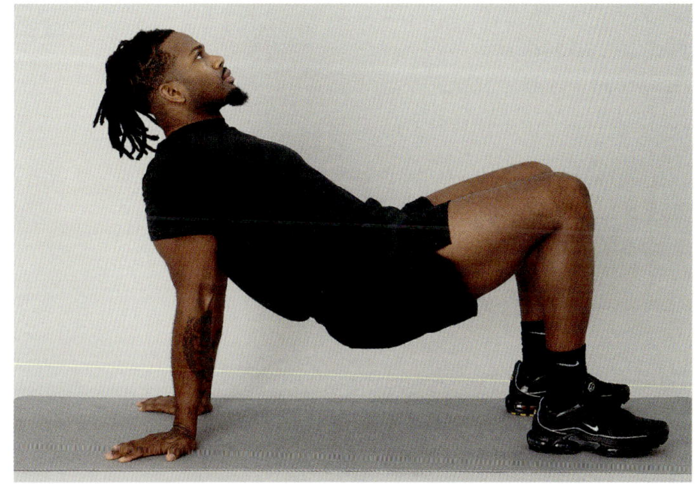

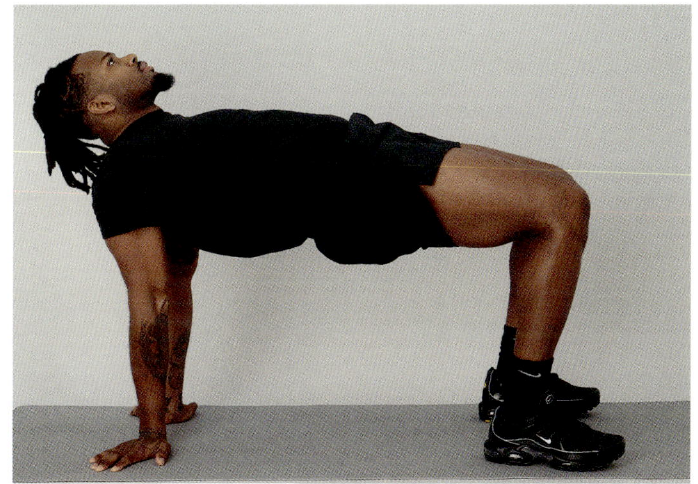

Side Plank with Hip Lifts

EQUIPMENT: Exercise mat or rug for support

2 SETS OF 12–20 REPS EACH SIDE

Starting position

Lie on your side, supporting yourself on your forearm, with legs straight.

The movement

Press into your forearm and feet to lift your hip off the mat. Pause for 1 second at the top before coming back down under control. Complete the same number of reps on each side.

Tip: Stagger your feet in front and back for additional support, or place your feet closer together, or stack them, to increase the difficulty.

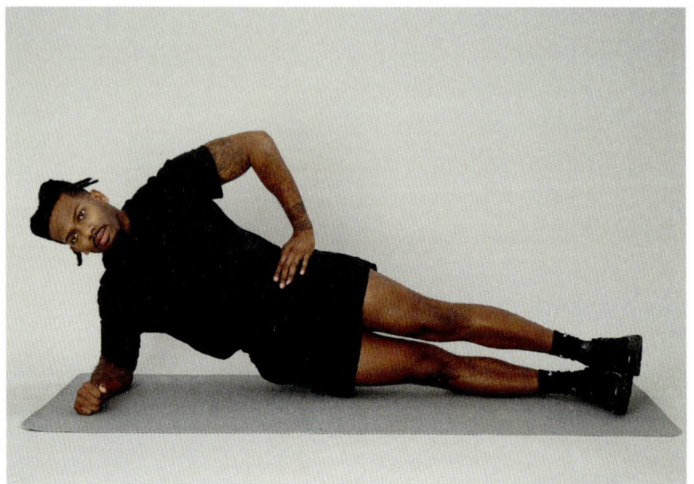

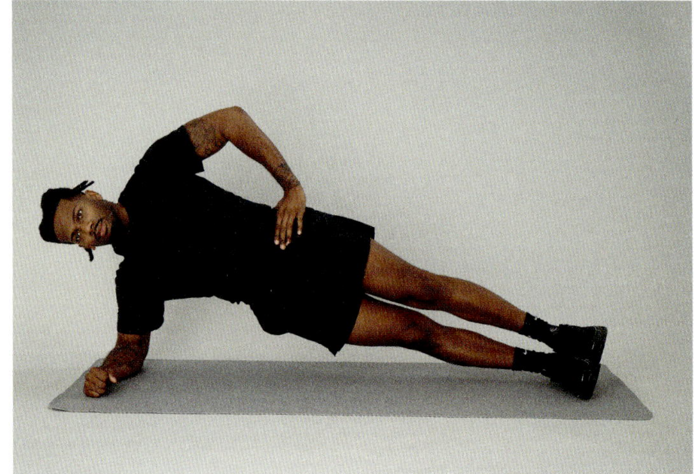

V-Sits

EQUIPMENT: Exercise mat or rug for support

2 SETS OF 12–16 REPS

Starting position
Lie on your back with legs straight, and place your hands in front of your face.

The movement
Contract all of the muscles along the front of your body to lift your legs and torso off the floor at the same time to form a V shape. Straighten your arms as you lift your legs, as if you're reaching for your toes. A curved back is okay; it helps engage the abdominals more.

Tip: Bend your knees, or keep your hands close to your chest to make the exercise easier.

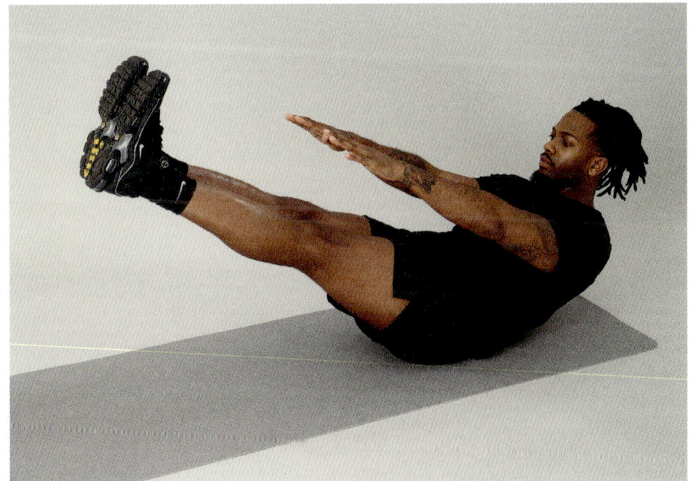

Conclusion

The single most important quality in developing longevity from your workout regimen is emphasizing control. Each exercise in this program requires a great deal of full-body control at all times. Each is meant to be practiced with an emphasis on controlling your movement and position in space. Avoid letting momentum or gravity have its way with you.

Enjoy what your body can do. Each workout is an opportunity to appreciate the control you have. This appreciation will inspire you to maintain and grow the specific qualities that contribute to your health and longevity.

As I stated at the start, nature works on the principle of "use it or lose it." It's intrinsic to continue using that which you value and appreciate. And the more you strive for physical control, the more you'll come to appreciate your physical abilities, which will motivate you to continue the cycle for a lifetime of strength and longevity.

That said, don't worry about doing everything perfectly or trying to optimize your program to the point of perfection. Fitness isn't an all-or-nothing situation where it's either perfectly effective or not effective at all. Your consistent action and mindful attention to your technique will place you firmly on the right path.

My grandfather (who was a prime example of strength and longevity) always said, "Play the cards that life deals you." We're all built differently, and we all face unique challenges. The best thing you can do is do the best you can with what you have. As you take advantage of the opportunity to continue learning, growing, and caring for your body, you can rest assured you're adding years to your life and life to your years.

SAMPLE SCHEDULE

SUN	MON	TUE	WED	THU	FRI	SAT

WORKOUT #1	WORKOUT #2	WORKOUT #3

SAMPLE SCHEDULE

SUN	MON	TUE	WED	THU	FRI	SAT

WORKOUT #1	WORKOUT #2	WORKOUT #3

Resources

Equipment

RESISTANCE BANDS AND DOOR ANCHORS

High-quality resistance bands and door anchors are recommended for scalable strength training, mobility work, and rehabilitation exercises. These tools are lightweight, portable, and adaptable to a wide range of fitness levels and training environments.

Supplier: Amazon ▪ https://a.co/d/b5seBAx

SUSPENSION TRAINING SYSTEMS

Suspension straps allow for bodyweight-based strength training that emphasizes core stability, balance, and functional movement patterns. They are particularly effective for developing total-body strength using minimal equipment.

Supplier: NOSSK Suspension Straps ▪ nossk.com

Professional Resources and Contact Information

RED DELTA PROJECT

The Red Delta Project is the author's platform, where you can find education, coaching, and training systems focused on intelligent strength development, biomechanics, and long-term physical resilience.

Website: reddeltaproject.com
Contact: reddeltaproject@gmail.com

Research and Evidence-Based Training

For readers interested in the scientific foundations of strength training and practical applications of current research, the following resource offers in-depth analysis and evidence-based recommendations:

Stronger by Science: strongerbyscience.com

Further Reading

Mobility Man by Al Kavadlo (ebook)
Old Man Strength by Al Kavadlo (ebook)
Overcoming Isometrics by Matt Schifferle
Strength Rules by Danny Kavadlo
Temple Maintenance with Resistance Bands by Michael Cook

Index

Acknowledgments

This book simply could not be possible without the long-term support and feedback of all of my friends, family, and clients. Their feedback and valuable insights about how to grow and improve through years of trial and error have helped me evolve as a coach to bring this program to you.

Special thanks to Mary, Seth, Melissa, Erika, and Robert for challenging me to look beyond my own nose to learn how to become the coach I am today.

About the Author

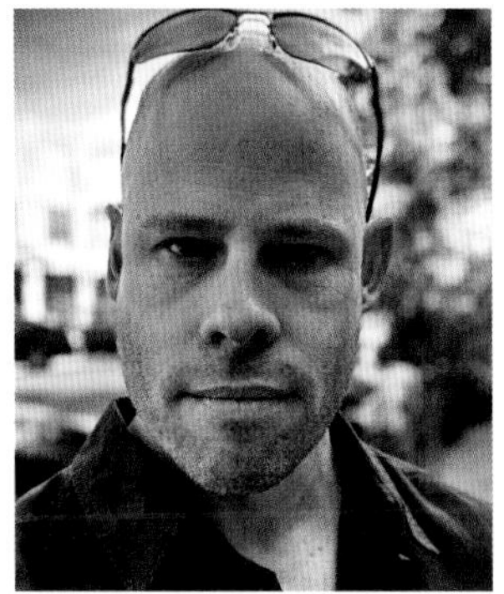

Matt Schifferle (shif-er-lee) is on a mission to help people break free from the fitness rat race and make the whole world stronger through calisthenics training. A fitness coach for more than two decades, he created Red Delta Project to empower people with more freedom and control over their health.

Matt works with a wide variety of clients in Denver, Colorado, where he's constantly testing his fundamental approach to fitness with a wide variety of clients and athletes. He is the author of over a dozen books, including *Grind Style Calisthenics, Micro Workouts, Smart Bodyweight Training*, and *Beautiful Strength*. Most days you can find Matt kicking back at one of the local brewpubs after a day of skiing or mountain biking.

Learn more about Matt and his fitness approach at reddeltaproject.com, and visit him on Instagram @red.delta.project.

About the Photographer

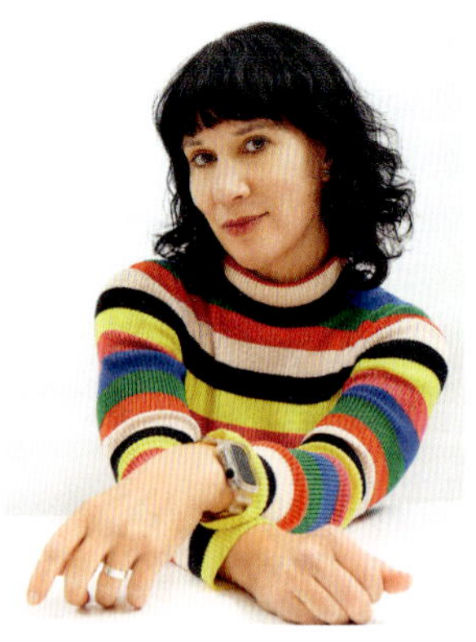

Jena Cumbo is a New York–based photographer and video maker specializing in fitness-, beauty-, and portrait-driven fashion lifestyle work.

She creates imagery that emphasizes movement, strength, and presence. Her work feels contemporary and body aware, with clean compositions and natural lighting that keep the focus on the subject. Shooting both stills and motion, she delivers polished yet approachable visuals that connect easily with today's audiences.

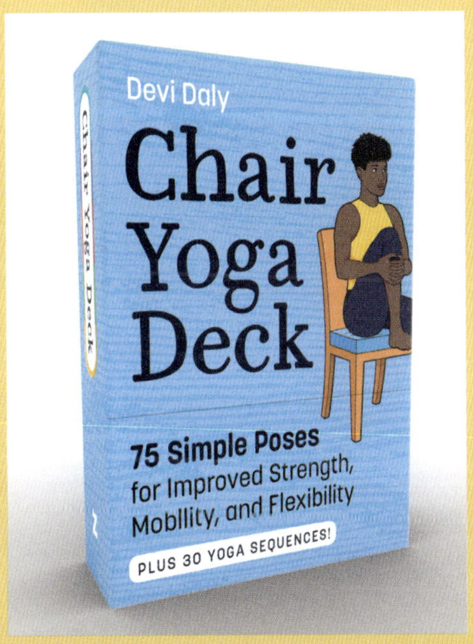

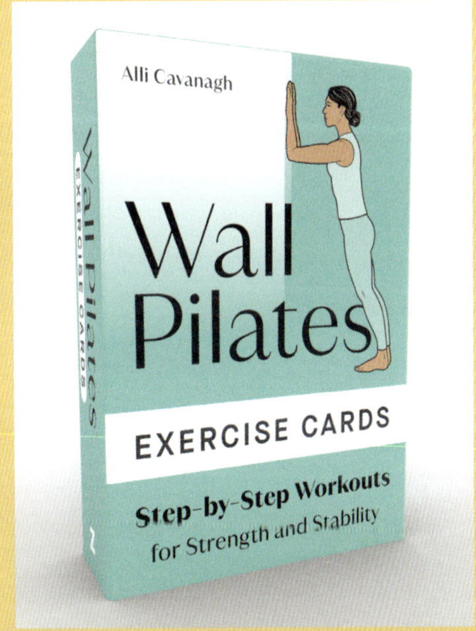

If you loved this book, expand your routine with
Chair Yoga and Wall Pilates decks—simple, effective ways to
boost mobility, stability, and total-body power anywhere.

Discover more at zeitgeistpublishing.com.

Hi there,

We hope you enjoyed *Strength Training for Longevity*. If you have any questions or concerns about your book, or have received a damaged copy, please contact customerservice@penguinrandomhouse.com. We're here and happy to help.

Also, please consider writing a review on your favorite retailer's website to let others know what you thought of the book!

Sincerely,
The Zeitgeist Team